KT-464-683

Fitness and Health

ISSUES

Volume 113

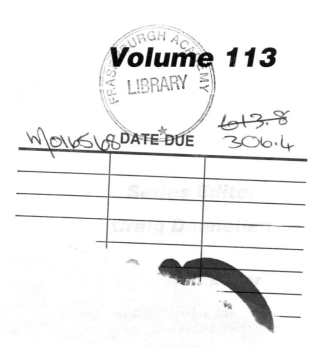
FRASERBURGH ACADEMY LIBRARY

DATE DUE

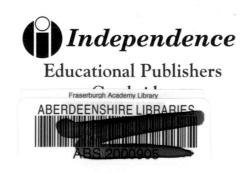
Independence
Educational Publishers

Fraserburgh Academy Library
ABERDEENSHIRE LIBRARIES

ABS2000905

First published by Independence
PO Box 295
Cambridge CB1 3XP
England

© Craig Donnellan 2006

Copyright
This book is sold subject to the condition that it shall not,
by way of trade or otherwise, be lent, resold, hired out or otherwise
circulated in any form of binding or cover other than that in which it
is published without the publisher's prior consent.

Photocopy licence
The material in this book is protected by copyright. However, the
purchaser is free to make multiple copies of particular articles for instructional
purposes for immediate use within the purchasing institution.
Making copies of the entire book is not permitted.

British Library Cataloguing in Publication Data
Fitness and Health – (Issues Series)
I. Donnellan, Craig II. Series
306.4'613

ISBN 1 86168 346 4

Printed in Great Britain
MWL Print Group Ltd

Layout by
Lisa Firth

Cover
The illustration on the front cover is by
Angelo Madrid.

CONTENTS

Chapter One: Our Fitness Problem

Chapter Two: Getting Fit

FRASERBURGH ACADEMY LIBRARY

Introduction

Fitness and Health is the one hundred and thirteenth volume in the **Issues** series. The aim of this series is to offer up-to-date information about important issues in our world.

Fitness and Health looks at Britain's fitness problem and how to get fit.

The information comes from a wide variety of sources and includes:
Government reports and statistics
Newspaper reports and features
Magazine articles and surveys
Website material
Literature from lobby groups
and charitable organisations.

It is hoped that, as you read about the many aspects of the issues explored in this book, you will critically evaluate the information presented. It is important that you decide whether you are being presented with facts or opinions. Does the writer give a biased or an unbiased report? If an opinion is being expressed, do you agree with the writer?

Fitness and Health offers a useful starting-point for those who need convenient access to information about the many issues involved. However, it is only a starting-point. At the back of the book is a list of organisations which you may want to contact for further information.

*****

90% of children 'set to be couch potatoes'

By Denis Campbell

Nine out of 10 schoolchildren are not doing enough exercise to ensure that they grow into healthy adults, according to a major new study.

Only 10 per cent of young people get the one hour a day of physical activity that ministers, health experts and scientists say is necessary.

The findings have sparked new fears that many young Britons are turning into 'couch potatoes' whose sedentary lifestyles mean they are much more likely to become obese in later life and suffer a whole range of diseases. They underline how age-old habits such as playing football in the street have been replaced by indoor pursuits involving computers and televisions.

When researchers monitored activity levels among 4,500 11-year-old pupils in the Bristol area using sophisticated motion sensors called 'accelerometers', they found that some did no exercise at all, only a few did the recommended daily hour, and most did some but not enough.

'Kids should be doing 60 minutes a day of moderate to vigorous exercise to be truly healthy and ensure their bones and cardio-vascular systems develop properly. But this study shows that most are not doing that', said Professor Chris Riddoch, head of the London Sports Institute at Middlesex University, who led the research. Riddoch is a government adviser on children's health and international expert on physical activity.

'Children are doing a lot of exercise such as walking, but just not enough vigorous stuff like running around and playing football. The fact that more and more of them are getting fatter shows that they aren't balancing the energy they take in from food by burning off calories through exercise', he added.

Recent Office of National Statistics figures showed that 22 per cent of boys and 28 per cent of girls aged two to 15 in England were overweight or obese, while a study last month said British children were the third fattest in the world after the US and Malta.

Experts in obesity said Riddoch's research, part of the Avon Longitudinal Study of Parents and Children, was alarming but inevitable.

'We live in a society where parents are too frightened to let their kids out to play, school playing fields have been sold off and streets are so packed with parked cars that youngsters have nowhere to kick a ball around even if they feel like it', said Neville Rigby of the International Obesity Task Force.

'We need to do nothing less than change the world they are growing up in. We have to create safer spaces for them to play in so they have an incentive to leave their keyboard behind and go outside, and reduce the amount of fatty and sugary foods they consume', added Rigby.

Dr Ian Campbell, chairman of the National Obesity Forum, said: 'If we want these trends to change we need to redesign our built environment to encourage walking and cycling, make it safe for children to be outdoors, and learn to eat together as families again in a non-rushed way.'

Campbell urged ministers to put money into promoting physical activity as a normal part of everyday life, and not just into sport.

Boys were much more likely than girls to do an hour a day, while children from lower socio-economic groups do more than peers from better-off backgrounds, according to Riddoch's survey.

The Department of Health declined to comment on Riddoch's findings, which he will present at next week's American College of Sports Medicine annual conference in Nashville, Tennessee. But a spokeswoman confirmed that the Chief Medical Officer's advice is that 'children and young people should achieve a total of at least 60 minutes of moderate-intensity physical activity each day'.

The Government's Physical Education School Sport and Club Links strategy was increasing the amount of PE and sport which pupils did in and out of school, she said.

■ This article first appeared in the *Observer*, 29 May 2005.

© *Guardian Newspapers Limited 2005*

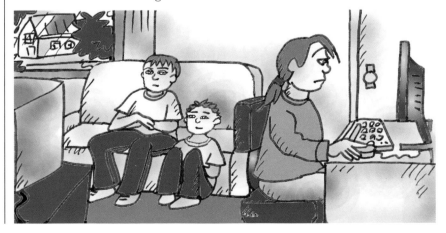

TV link to obese children

Information from *Which?* magazine

The amount of time kids spend watching televison is a key factor in childhood obesity, a new study suggests.

Scientists in New Zealand monitored more than 1,000 youngsters up until the age of 26 to see whether there was a link between their weight and the amount of TV they watched.

The research team found that their viewing habits had more effect on their body mass index (BMI) – a measurement which calculates weight compared to height – than either what they ate or how much they exercised.

Which? believes this link illustrates the urgent need for tighter controls on the TV advertising of junk food during children's viewing hours.

'While there are many barriers to healthy eating the effect of TV advertising on children's food choices cannot be ignored,' said *Which?* food campaigner Miranda Watson.

'We are calling on the communications regulator Ofcom to tackle this problem by restricting foods high in fat, sugar and salt from being advertised during children's viewing times.'

At various times during the study, the parents, and later the children themselves, recorded how long the youngsters watched television each week.

Researchers found that teenagers aged 13 to 15 watched an average of 24.6 hours per week. Those who watched more TV had a higher BMI.

The study, published in the *International Journal of Obesity*, found that over two-fifths of people who were overweight or obese by the age of 26 had watched the most TV as a child.
14 September 2005

■ The above information is reprinted with kind permission from *Which?* Visit www.which.co.uk for more information.

© *Which?*

How many people are obese?

Information from Weight Concern

Worldwide obesity epidemic

■ Globally more than 1 billion adults are overweight and 300 million adults are obese. Approximately 17.6 million children are overweight worldwide.
(*Source: www.who.int*)

■ Contrary to popular belief, the obesity epidemic is not just a problem in developed countries, the number of individuals who are overweight or obese is also increasing in developing countries.

■ In Sub-Saharan Africa, a place that is associated with famine and malnutrition, 12% of women are overweight.
(*Source: www.iotf.org*)

Obesity in the United Kingdom

■ In the UK, the number of people who are overweight or obese has been rising at an alarming rate over the last 20 years.

■ In 1980, 6% of men and 8% of women were obese (a body mass index above 30 kg/m^2) compared with 22.1% of men and 22.8% of women who were obese in 2002.

■ 43.4% of men and 33.7% of women were overweight in 2002 (a body mass index of 25-29.9 kg/m^2).

■ Based on population data from 2002, 11.1 million men and 9.0 million women living in the UK are overweight and 11.8 million people are obese.

■ The levels of overweight and obese have also been rising in children. In 2002, one in 20 boys and one in 15 girls aged 2-15 years were obese.

■ Overall, over one in five boys and one in four girls are either overweight or obese.
(*Source: Health Survey for England 2002 and Health Select Committee report on Obesity May 2004*)

■ If these trends continue, it has been estimated that by 2020, one-third of all adults and 50% of children in the UK will be obese.
(*Source: Health Select Committee report on Obesity May 2004*)

■ The above information is reprinted with kind permission from Weight Concern. Visit www.shape-up.org for more information or see page 41 for their address details.

© *Weight Concern*

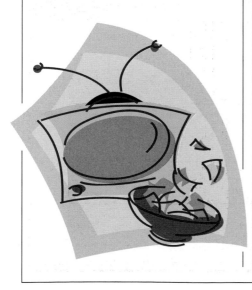

Obesity among children under 11

A summary

This report presents key information about obesity among children aged under 11 living in England, based on data from the Health Survey for England. It is intended to support the development of an evidence-based approach to prevention, management and treatment of obesity in children.

- Between 1995 and 2003, the prevalence of obesity among children aged 2 to 10 rose from 9.9% to 13.7%.
- The percentage of children aged 2 to 10 who were overweight (including those who were obese) rose from 22.7% in 1995 to 27.7% in 2003.
- Overall, levels of obesity were similar for both boys and girls aged 2 to 10. For boys, obesity rose from 9.6% in 1995 to 14.9% in 2003, for girls obesity rose from 10.3% in 1995 to 12.5% in 2003.
- Between 1995 and 2003, levels of obesity rose among children aged 2 to 10. However, increases in obesity prevalence were most significant among older children aged 8 to 10, rising from 11.2% in 1995 to 16.5% in 2003.
- Obesity prevalence among children aged 2 to 10 varied according to region and area type. Obesity levels were lowest in Yorkshire and the Humber (11.4%) and the South East (13.4%) and highest in the North East (18.3%) and London (18.2%) in 2001 and 2002. Furthermore, obesity was higher among children living in inner-city areas than among children living in all other types of area.
- In 2001 and 2002, levels of obesity for children aged 2 to 10 differed between various socio-demographic groups. For example, children living within households with the lowest levels of household income had higher rates of obesity than children from households with the highest levels of household income (15.8% compared with 13.3%).

Increases in obesity prevalence were most significant among older children aged 8 to 10, rising from 11.2% in 1995 to 16.5% in 2003

The same pattern was evident within different levels of area deprivation. Levels of obesity were 5 percentage points higher among children living within the most deprived areas (16.4%) than the least deprived areas (11.2%). Within socio-economic group (analysed using the National Statistics Social-Economic Classification, a classification similar to social class), 17.1% of children within semi-routine and routine households were obese compared with 12.4% of those from managerial and professional households.

- 19.8% of children living in households where both parents were either overweight or obese were themselves obese compared with 6.7% of children living in households where neither parents were overweight or obese and 8.4% of children living in households where one of the two parents was overweight or obese.
- This report uses the UK National Body Mass Index (BMI) percentile classification to describe childhood overweight and obesity among children aged 2-10. Explanation of this measure and details of how obesity and overweight are categorised are given in the technical annex of this report.

- The above information is the summary of the report *Obesity among children under 11*, published April 2005, from the Department of Health. Visit www.dh.gov.uk to view the full report or for more information.

© *Crown copyright*

Childhood obesity trends

Trends in overweight and obesity prevalence among children (aged 2-10 with valid BMI), by survey year (1995-2003)

Source: 'Obesity among children under 11', Dept. of Health. Crown copyright.

Childhood obesity

Britain's kids need food for thought

Exclusive consumer research from Mintel's first comprehensive report into childhood obesity names a staggering one in three (33%) Mums and Dads as 'Relaxed Parents', who take little interest in their children's eating habits. This amounts to some 5.3 million parents, making 'Relaxed Parents' the largest group of Mums and Dads in Britain today. But when it comes to children's diet, it is clear that Mum does know best, with just a quarter (27%) of Mums falling into this group, compared to as many as two in five (41%) Dads.

While in general, three-quarters (75%) of parents with children under 16 claim that they try to ensure their kids eat a healthy diet, only just over half (54%) say that they try to actually educate their children about healthy eating. What is more, a similar proportion (just 51%) mention putting into place any specific course of action such as avoiding too much sugar, while just two in five (42%) avoid giving kids high fat foods.

'Over the past few months there has been considerable media coverage about the problems of child obesity. But the time has come to take action and to move away from simply who is to blame. Although messages about the importance of leading a healthy life seem to be getting through, too many parents are still unsure about how to actually put a healthy diet into practice. Clearly parents need practical suggestions, such as how to ensure their child eats five portions of fruit and veg a day, to make leading a healthy life as easy as possible,' comments Maria Elustondo, senior market analyst at Mintel.

Parents also need to realise that weight gain is not just down to the child's diet. Indeed, weight gain amongst Britain's children is often related to their increasingly sedentary lifestyle, with many children spending a large amount of time slumped in front of the television or playing on computers and game consoles.

'Clearly children need to be encouraged to become more active as well as to have a healthier diet. But the health education process is not an area open solely to the public sector. Indeed, there are plenty of further opportunities for the private sector to get involved and provide help in this area. Companies could look into introducing easy-to-follow books, videos and counselling, while private health clubs could benefit from focusing on developing family-based exercise programmes,' comments Maria Elustondo.

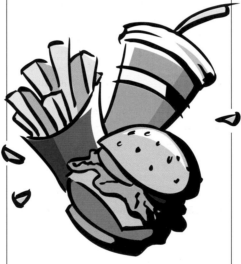

The remainder of parents are 'Indulging Parents' (17%), who give their children what they want when it comes to food, whether it is healthy or not, 'Worrying Parents' (21%), who are concerned about their children's weight as well as their sugar and fat intake and 'Controlling Parents' (29%), who try and ensure their children eat a healthy diet.

Kids – concentrate on curbing those carbs

The vast majority (72%) of 11-16-year-olds know that it is important to eat a balanced diet, but many do not seem to be putting this knowledge into practice. Despite significant drops since 2001 almost seven in ten (67%) still often eat between meals, and over half (53%) claim to eat whatever they like.

There is obviously a strong carbohydrate element to children's diet these days, with bread (85%), fruit (82%), biscuits (80%), cereals (78%) and tomato ketchup (78%) named as the top five foods for Britain's seven- to 16-year-old children. And while it is encouraging to see that as many as eight in ten (82%) do eat fruit, it is of some concern that far fewer, at just seven in ten (69%), eat vegetables.

When it comes to eating between meals, the situation is equally as worrying, with just one out of the top five snacks of choice proving to be a healthier option. The top choice is potato crisps (41%), followed by chocolate (39%), then comes fruit (35%), sweets (29%) and sweet biscuits (22%).

'Children need to be educated on the benefits of a healthy diet for themselves, in order to understand how it affects their lifestyles. This could be done by marketing certain foods as "beauty foods", which are good for healthy skin, hair and nails, or "sports fuel". The main point being that they understand how eating a healthy diet and taking regular exercise, can have a positive impact on their life and what they enjoy doing,' explains Maria.

Sugar and spice and all things nice?

Girls are much more interested than boys in healthy eating, with three-quarters (76%) of girls understanding the importance of eating a balanced diet, compared to fewer than seven in ten (68%) boys. Girls are also more likely to mention the practical statements such as not eating 'too many sweets' (51% of girls vs 43% of boys) and 'trying not to eat too much' (54% of girls vs 43% of boys).

But at the other end of the spectrum there are growing concerns about children becoming obsessed with their weight at a young age. Worryingly, as many as one in three (33%) children say that they often try to lose weight – whether they need to or not – and a similar proportion (32%) eat when they are sad. Three in ten (30%) also say that they sometimes feel guilty about eating.

Girls (44%) are almost twice as likely as boys (23%) to be trying to lose weight, and are also more likely to feel guilty about eating (41% of girls vs 20% of boys) and to comfort eat (41% of girls vs 23% of boys).

About Mintel

Mintel is a worldwide leader of competitive media, product and consumer intelligence. For more than 30 years, Mintel has provided key insight into leading global trends. With offices in Chicago, London, Belfast and Sydney, Mintel's innovative product line provides unique data that have a direct impact on client success. For more information on Mintel, please visit their website at www.mintel.com.
June 2005

© *Mintel*

Children's diets

Information from Weight Loss Resources

This month (July 2005), the papers have been packed with news about school dinners and children's diets. In the hit Channel 4 show, *Jamie's School Dinners*, TV chef Jamie Oliver showed the nation exactly what many British children were being fed for lunch at school – and it wasn't good news! Most were filling up on junk food like chips, pizzas, nuggets and burgers, and were horrified at the thought of eating fresh food and vegetables. But worse still, catering staff simply didn't have enough money or resources to provide better quality lunches.

The medical director of the British Heart Foundation warned that many obese teenagers could face heart attacks in their 40s

---

Now, after weeks of campaigning to end school junk food, Jamie is delighted the government has finally agreed to spend a minimum of 50p a day on ingredients for each child in primary school education – and 60p for those in secondary schools – instead of the average of 37p. In addition, more money will be available for training cooks and a School Food Trust will be set up to advise on how to make meals healthier and tastier. Meanwhile, the Labour Party has pledged to ban junk food adverts during children's TV if

By Juliette Kellow BSc SRD WLR Dietitian

food companies don't take the plunge themselves.

Many experts agree the move to improve children's diets couldn't come soon enough. In February, the medical director of the British Heart Foundation made one of the starkest predictions yet, warning that many obese teenagers could face heart attacks in their 40s. And only last month, official government figures showed that hospital admissions for obese children were up almost a third from last year, indicating that overweight youngsters are placing an increasing strain on the health service.

But it's not just children's health that's affected by diet. As *Jamie's School Dinners* showed, if children eat healthily, their behaviour and performance at school is also likely to improve. In March this year, government research showed exactly this. They found that primary schools who belonged to the government's national healthy schools programme – where children are encouraged to have a healthier lifestyle – outperformed those that didn't belong to the programme in national tests for English, Maths and Science.

Weight Loss Resources says...

Currently, 8.5 per cent of six-year-olds and 15 per cent of 15-year-olds are obese and are setting themselves up for a range of health problems

when they're older, including type 2 diabetes, heart disease, certain cancers, high blood pressure and joint and back problems to name just a few. It's good news then, that as a nation, we're finally beginning to recognise the importance of feeding our children a healthier diet. The challenge is now to ensure that parents, schools, food manufacturers, government and the health service work together to achieve the best results possible.

Juliette's tips

One of the most important things we can do as parents is to provide our children with healthy meals and snacks. But it's also important to talk to children about food and encourage them to cook or help out in the kitchen. Young children, in particular, love cooking and are far more likely to eat something they've made themselves, so get them involved in making simple recipes like fruit smoothies, or filled pitta breads. Children also learn by example – you can't expect a child to eat loads of fruit and veg if you never touch the stuff yourself – so make it your mission to ensure the whole family has a healthy diet. It's not just your children who will benefit – your waistline will love you for it too!
20 July 2005

■ The above information is reprinted with kind permission from Weight Loss Resources. Visit www.weightlossresources.co.uk for more information.

© *Weight Loss Resources*

Call for Jamie Oliver of the gym

Schools need a Jamie Oliver of PE to tackle childhood obesity, it has been claimed

Developed countries need to take urgent action to stem the growing numbers of fat children, Colin Boreham, professor of sport and exercise science at the University of Ulster, has told a World Health Organisation (WHO) symposium. The solution must include concerted promotion of physical exercise among school pupils, he said.

Professor Boreham, who has represented Britain in athletics at the Olympics, said: 'Rising levels of childhood obesity are possibly the most pressing public health concern in developed countries like the UK and USA.

'If current trends continue, a majority of children aged 10 to 15 are predicted to be overweight. That cannot be allowed to happen, because being overweight in childhood has both immediate and long-term health implications.'

Prof Boreham, an expert on obesity, was asked by the WHO to contribute his expertise to a conference of global analysts in Japan who are to draw up a set of guidelines for combating the condition in children.

'If current trends continue, a majority of children aged 10 to 15 are predicted to be overweight'

Childhood obesity has only been recognised in the past 20 years, and Northern Ireland is one of only a few places in the world where children's weight has been studied over a 10-year period – in the Young Hearts project at the University of Ulster.

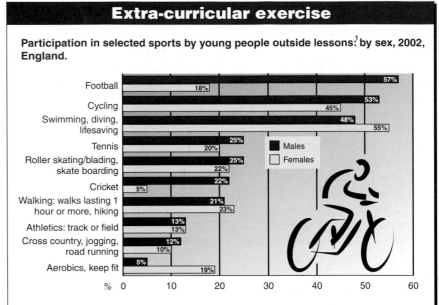

Extra-curricular exercise

Participation in selected sports by young people outside lessons:[1] by sex, 2002, England.

- Football — Males 57%, Females 18%
- Cycling — Males 53%, Females 45%
- Swimming, diving, lifesaving — Males 48%, Females 55%
- Tennis — Males 25%, Females 20%
- Roller skating/blading, skate boarding — Males 25%, Females 22%
- Cricket — Males 22%, Females 5%
- Walking: walks lasting 1 hour or more, hiking — Males 21%, Females 23%
- Athletics: track or field — Males 13%, Females 13%
- Cross country, jogging, road running — Males 12%, Females 10%
- Aerobics, keep fit — Males 5%, Females 19%

% 0 10 20 30 40 50 60

1. Those aged 6 to 16 participating at least 10 times in the 12 months leading up to the survey.

Source: Sports England/MORI. Crown copyright.

'We have very good objective evidence of children having become fatter over a 10-year period,' Prof Boreham said.

Contributory factors include lifestyle changes such as the growth of indoor pursuits – computer-based activities, for example – at the expense of the outdoor games of the past.

The rise in consumption of processed foods and the increasing popularity of eating out – and consuming richer foods in greater quantities – was the other key factor.

Professor Boreham told the Kobe conference that school was the ideal setting for instigating positive change. 'What we need is an integrated approach that links many aspects of child behaviour both inside and outside the school.

'We have to look to legislation; we have to change the school curriculum and the school environment. We need an approach that looks at physical activity, including even the school transportation programme.'

Many European schools promoted cycling to school, he said. But, looking at the UK, he said: 'How many schools here would be prepared to promote cycling to school – and how many even have a school bikeshed any more?'

Citing the results of the Young Hearts study, he said governments and society more broadly must act quickly to change attitudes towards the quality and quantity of food – and the need for exercise.

'It's remarkable what individuals can achieve,' he said, adding: 'Almost overnight, Jamie Oliver was responsible for raising awareness about the quality of school meals, to the extent where physical action became a political imperative.

'If we have to have a Jamie Oliver for physical education as well, then so be it!'

Printed in the Guardian, 14 July 2005.
© The Press Association

Avoiding childhood obesity

Information from BUPA

Children have high energy requirements because they are growing. A varied and nutritious diet is essential for their development. However, like adults, if they take in more energy in the form of food than they use up, the extra energy is stored in their bodies as fat.

It is estimated that up to 15% of children in the UK are overweight or obese.

It's a serious problem

Children who are overweight tend to grow up into adults who are overweight. They therefore have a higher risk of developing serious health problems in later life, including heart attack and stroke, type 2 diabetes, bowel cancer, and high blood pressure. The risk of health problems increases the more overweight a person becomes.

Being overweight as a child can also cause psychological distress. Teasing about their appearance affects children's confidence and self-esteem and can lead to isolation and depression.

The number of overweight and obese children in the UK has risen steadily over the past 20 years. This is now a major health concern.

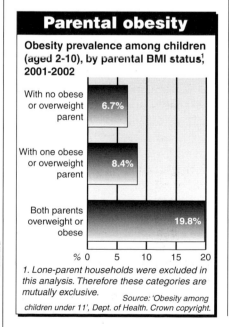

Parental obesity

Obesity prevalence among children (aged 2-10), by parental BMI status[1], 2001-2002

With no obese or overweight parent: 6.7%

With one obese or overweight parent: 8.4%

Both parents overweight or obese: 19.8%

% 0 5 10 15 20

1. Lone-parent households were excluded in this analysis. Therefore these categories are mutually exclusive.

Source: 'Obesity among children under 11', Dept. of Health. Crown copyright.

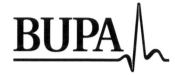

feel better

Why are more children overweight?

Very few children become overweight because of an underlying medical problem. Children are more likely to be overweight if their parents are obese. But genetic factors are thought to be less significant than the fact that families tend to share eating and activity habits.

In other words, most children put on excess weight because their lifestyles include an unhealthy diet and a lack of physical activity.

It is certainly easier than ever before for children to become overweight. High-calorie foods, such as fast food and confectionery, are abundant, relatively cheap and heavily promoted specifically at children.

Exercise is no longer a regular part of everyone's day – some children never walk or cycle to school, or play any kind of sport. And it is not unusual for children to spend hours in front of a television or computer. The National Diet and Nutrition Survey (2000) found that 40-69% of children over the age of six spend less than the recommended minimum of one hour a day doing moderate intensity physical activity.

What is a healthy weight for a child?

Parents may find it difficult to tell whether their child has temporary 'puppy fat' or is genuinely overweight. In adults, a simple formula (the body mass index, or BMI) is used to work out whether a person is the right weight for their height.

However, BMI alone is not an appropriate measure for children – it has to be used alongside charts that

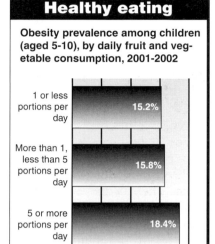

Healthy eating

Obesity prevalence among children (aged 5-10), by daily fruit and vegetable consumption, 2001-2002

1 or less portions per day: 15.2%

More than 1, less than 5 portions per day: 15.8%

5 or more portions per day: 18.4%

% 0 5 10 15 20

Source: 'Obesity among children under 11', Dept. of Health. Crown copyright.

take into account the child's rate of growth, sex and age – and is best interpreted with the help of your GP, health visitor, practice nurse or dietitian.

It is possible to measure the proportion of a child's weight that is made up of fat. Generally speaking, a child's weight is classed as obese when their body weight is more than 25% fat in boys and 32% in girls.

Maintaining a healthy weight

Expert advice is that most children who are overweight should not be encouraged to actually lose weight. Instead they are encouraged to maintain their weight, so they gradually 'grow into it' as they get taller.

Children should never be put on a weight-loss diet without medical advice as this can affect their growth. Unregulated dieting – particularly in teenage girls – is thought to lead to the development of eating disorders.

No drug treatment has been proven effective in the treatment of weight problems in children.

Helping children to achieve and maintain a healthy weight involves a threefold approach that encourages them to:

- eat a healthy, well-balanced diet
- make changes to eating habits
- reduce physical inactivity.

The good news is that all the evidence shows that it is much easier to change a child's eating and exercise habits than it is to alter an adult's.

A healthy well-balanced diet

Parents concerned about their child's weight should encourage a variety of fresh, nutritious foods in his or her diet.

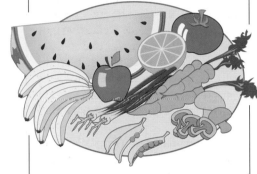

- Starchy foods, which are rich in 'complex carbohydrates', are bulky relative to the amount of calories they contain. This makes them filling and nutritious. Sources such as bread, potatoes, pasta, rice and chapatti should provide half the energy in a child's diet.
- Instead of high-fat foods like chocolate, biscuits, cakes and crisps, try healthier alternatives such as fresh fruit, crusty bread or crackers.
- Try to grill or bake foods instead of frying. Burgers, fish fingers and sausages are just as tasty when grilled, but have a lower fat content. Oven chips are lower in fat than fried chips.
- Avoid fizzy drinks that are high in sugar. Substitute them with fresh juices diluted with water or sugar-free alternatives.
- A healthy breakfast of a low-sugar cereal (e.g. wholemeal wheat biscuits) with milk, plus a piece of fruit is a good start to the day.
- Instead of sweets, offer dried fruit or tinned fruit in natural juice. Frozen yoghurt is an alternative to ice cream. Bagels are an alternative to doughnuts.

Changes to eating habits

- Try to set a good example with your own eating habits.

- Provide meals and snacks at regular times to prevent 'grazing' throughout the day.
- Don't allow your children to eat while watching TV or doing homework.
- Make mealtimes an occasion by eating as a family group as often as possible.
- Encourage children to 'listen to their tummies' and eat when they are hungry rather than out of habit.
- Teach children to chew food more slowly and savour the food. They will feel fuller more quickly and be less likely to overeat at mealtimes.
- Do not keep lots of high-fat, high-sugar snack foods in the house.
- Do not make outings for fast foods part of the weekly routine.
- Try to get children involved in preparing food as this will make them more aware of what they are eating.
- When children who need to improve their eating habits are old enough, it may help them to keep a food diary, recording what and when they eat. It's important to be aware of snacking 'danger times' and find strategies to divert attention away from food, or towards a healthier option.

Physical activity

Doctors recommend a gradual increase in physical activity, such as brisk walking, to at least an hour a day.

- Encourage walking to places such as school and the shops, rather than always jumping in the car.
- Suggest going to the park for a kick around with a football, or a game of rounders, cricket or frisbee.
- Visit a local leisure centre to investigate sports and team activities to get involved in.
- Make exercise into a treat by taking special trips to an adventure play park or an ice skating rink, for example. Involve the whole family in bike rides, swimming and in-line skating.
- When it is safe to do so, teach your child to ride a bike.

Reducing physical inactivity

'Physical inactivity' includes pastimes such as watching TV or playing computer games. These should be reduced to no more than two hours a day or an average of 14 hours a week.

Encourage children to be selective about what they watch, concentrate only on the programmes they really enjoy.

Food can take on emotional significance when used to comfort or reward children

---

The emotional factors

Food can take on emotional significance when used to comfort or reward children.

- Do not use food to comfort a child – give attention, listening and hugs instead.
- Avoid using food as a reward as this can reinforce the idea of food as a source of comfort. Instead of having a fast-food meal to celebrate a good school report, for example, buy a gift, go to the cinema, or have a friend to stay overnight.

Prevention

- Studies show that breastfeeding a baby, even if only for a short period of time, may reduce the risk of obesity in later life.
- Parents who enjoy a healthy diet with plenty of fresh fruit and vegetables set a good example for their children. As children grow older they tend to stick to the eating pattern that has been established at home.

Further information

- British Nutrition Foundation www.nutrition.org.uk
- Food Standards Agency www.foodstandards.gov.uk/healthiereating

- The above information is reprinted with kind permission from BUPA, excluding any accompanying illustrations, diagrams and graphs. Visit www.bupa.co.uk/health for more information or see page 41 for their address details.

© BUPA

Obesity

Information from KidsHealth

The most important part of being a normal weight isn't looking a certain way – it's feeling good and staying healthy. Having too much body fat can be harmful to the body in many ways.

The number of people who are obese is rising. About 1.2 billion people in the world are overweight and at least 300 million of them are obese, even though obesity is one of the 10 most preventable health risks

The good news is that it's never too late to make changes in eating and exercise habits to control your weight, and those changes don't have to be as big as you might think. So if you or someone you know is obese or overweight, this article can give you information and tips for dealing with the problem by adopting a healthier lifestyle.

What is obesity?

Being obese and being overweight are not exactly the same thing. An obese person has a large amount of extra body fat, not just a few extra pounds. People who are obese are very overweight and at risk for serious health problems.

To determine if someone is obese, doctors and other health care professionals often use a measurement called body mass index (BMI). First, a doctor measures a person's height and weight. Then the doctor uses these numbers to calculate another number, the BMI.

Once the doctor has calculated a child's or teen's BMI, he or she will plot this number on a specific chart to see how it compares to other people of the same age and gender.

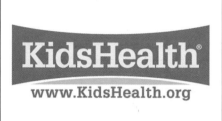

www.KidsHealth.org

A person with a BMI above the 95th percentile (meaning the BMI is greater than that of 95% of people of the same age and gender) is generally considered overweight. A person with a BMI between the 85th and 95th percentiles typically is considered at risk for overweight. Obesity is the term used for extreme overweight. There are some exceptions to this formula, though. For instance, someone who is very muscular (like a bodybuilder) may have a high BMI without being obese because the excess weight is from extra muscle, not fat.

What causes obesity?

People gain weight when the body takes in more calories than it burns off. Those extra calories are stored as fat. The amount of weight gain that leads to obesity doesn't happen in a few weeks or months. Because being obese is more than just being a few pounds overweight, people who are obese have usually been getting more calories than they need for years.

Genes – small parts of the DNA that people inherit from their parents and that determine traits like hair or eye colour – can play an important role in this weight gain. Some of your genes tell your body how to metabolise food and how to use extra calories or stored fat. Some people burn calories faster or slower than others do because of their genes.

Obesity can run in families, but just how much is due to genes is hard to determine. Many families eat the same foods, have the same habits (like snacking in front of the TV), and tend to think alike when it comes

to weight issues (like urging children to eat a lot at dinner so they can grow 'big and strong'). All of these situations can contribute to weight gain, so it can be difficult to figure out if a person is born with a tendency to be obese or overweight or learns eating and exercise habits that lead to weight gain. In most cases, weight problems arise from a combination of habits and genetic factors. Certain illnesses, like thyroid gland problems or unusual genetic disorders, are uncommon causes for people gaining weight.

Sometimes emotions can fuel obesity as well. People tend to eat more when they are upset, anxious, sad, stressed out, or even bored. Then after they eat too much, they may feel bad about it and eat more to deal with those bad feelings, creating a tough cycle to break.

One of the most important factors in weight gain is a sedentary lifestyle. People are much less active today than they used to be, with televisions, computers, and video games filling their spare time. Cars dominate our lives, and fewer people walk or ride bikes to get somewhere. As lives become busier, there is less time to cook healthy meals, so more and more people eat at restaurants, grab takeout food, or buy quick foods at the grocery store or food market to heat up at home. All of these can contain lots more fat and calories than meals prepared from fresh foods at home.

Who is at risk for becoming obese?

The number of people who are obese is rising. About 1.2 billion people in the world are overweight and at least 300 million of them are obese, even though obesity is one of the 10 most preventable health risks, according to the World Health Organization. In the United States, more than 97 million adults – that's more than half – are overweight and almost one in five adults is obese. Among teenagers and kids 6 years and older, more than 15% are overweight – that's more than three times the number of young people who were overweight in the 1970s. At least 300,000 deaths every year in the United States can be linked to obesity.

In the United States, women are slightly more at risk for becoming obese than men. Race and ethnicity also can be factors – in adolescents, obesity is more common among Mexican Americans and African Americans.

How can obesity affect your health?

Obesity is bad news for both body and mind. Not only does it make a person feel tired and uncomfortable, it can wear down joints and put extra stress on other parts of the body. When a person is carrying extra weight, it's harder to keep up with friends, play sports, or just walk between classes at school. It is also associated with breathing problems such as asthma and sleep apnoea and problems with hips and knee joints that may require surgery.

There can be more serious consequences as well. Obesity in young people can cause illnesses that once were thought to be problems only for adults, such as hypertension (high blood pressure), high cholesterol levels, liver disease, and type 2 diabetes, a disease in which the body has trouble converting food to energy, resulting in high blood sugar levels. As they get older, people who are obese are more likely to develop heart disease, congestive heart failure, bladder problems, and, in women, problems with the reproductive system. Obesity also can lead to stroke, greater risk for certain cancers such as breast or colon cancer, and even death.

In addition to other potential problems, people who are obese are more likely to be depressed. That can start a vicious cycle: when people are overweight, they may feel sad or even angry and eat to make themselves feel better. Then they feel worse for eating again. And when someone's feeling depressed, that person is less likely to go out and exercise.

How can you avoid becoming overweight or obese?

The best way to avoid these health problems is to maintain a healthy weight. And the keys to healthy weight are regular exercise and good eating habits.

To stay active, try to exercise 30 to 60 minutes every day. Your exercise doesn't have to be hard core, either. Walking, swimming, and stretching are all good ways to burn calories and help you stay fit. Try these activities to get moving:

- Go outside for a walk.
- Take the stairs instead of the elevator.
- Walk or bike to places (such as school or a friend's house) instead of driving.
- If you have to drive somewhere, park farther away than you need to and walk the extra distance.
- Tackle those household chores, such as vacuuming, washing the car, or cleaning the bathroom – they all burn calories.
- Alternate activities so you don't get bored: try running, biking, skating – the possibilities are endless.
- Limit your time watching TV or playing video games; even reading a book burns more energy.
- Go dancing – it can burn more than 300 calories an hour!

Eating well doesn't mean dieting over and over again to lose a few pounds. Instead, try to make healthy choices every day:

- Soft drinks, fruit juices, and sports drinks are loaded with sugar; drink fat-free or low-fat milk or water instead.
- Eat at least five servings of fruit and vegetables a day.
- Avoid fast-food restaurants. If you can't, try to pick healthier choices like grilled chicken or salads, and stick to regular servings – don't supersize!
- If you want a snack, try carrot sticks, a piece of fruit, or a piece of whole-grain toast instead of processed foods like chips and crackers, which can be loaded with fat and calories.
- Eat when you're hungry, not when you're bored or because you can't think of anything else to do.

- Eat a healthy breakfast every day.
- Don't eat meals or snacks while watching TV because you'll probably end up eating more than you intend to.
- Pay attention to the portion sizes of what you eat.

What can you do if you are overweight or obese?

Before you start trying to lose weight, talk to a doctor, a parent, or a registered dietitian. With their help, you can come up with a safe plan, based on eating well and exercising. Remember that teenagers need to keep eating regularly. Don't starve yourself because you won't get the nutrients you need to grow and develop normally.

You may also want to keep a food and activity journal. Keep track of what you eat, when you exercise, and how you feel. Changes can take time, but seeing your progress in writing will help you stick to your plan. You might also want to consider attending a support group; check your local hospital or the health section of a newspaper for groups that meet near you. Above all, surround yourself with friends and family who will be there for you and help you tackle these important changes in your life.

- This information was provided by KidsHealth, one of the largest resources online for medically reviewed health information for parents, kids and teens. For more articles like this one, visit their websites at www.teenshealth.org or www.kidshealth.org

© 1995-2005. The Nemours Foundation

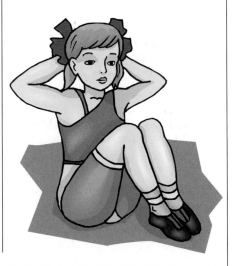

Obesity: the scale of the problem

Information from the Association for the Study of Obesity

Obesity as a global problem

The number of people who are obese is rising rapidly throughout the world, making obesity one of the fastest developing public health problems. The World Health Organization has described the problem of obesity as a 'worldwide epidemic'. It is estimated that around 1 billion people worldwide are overweight, of which 300 million are clinically obese (WHO, 2003).

> *The World Health Organization has described the problem of obesity as a 'worldwide epidemic'*

The USA has a particularly high prevalence of obesity. On average, over one-third of the adult population are obese, rising to more than 50% in some ethnic subgroups. Although the UK lags behind the USA, the rate of change is very similar to the USA and this offers a frightening insight into the potential scale of the problem unless adequate strategies are adopted now to both prevent and treat obesity.

Classification of obesity

Obesity is used to describe an excess of body fat to the extent to which it can cause ill-health. There are two methods for defining if an adult is overweight or obese.

1. The Body Mass Index (BMI)

The BMI is a tool for indicating weight status in adults. It is a measure of weight for height. This is defined as weight in kilograms divided by the height, in metres, squared:

$$\text{BMI (Kg/m}^2\text{)} = \frac{\text{WEIGHT (kg)}}{\text{HEIGHT (m)}^2}$$

ASSOCIATION FOR THE STUDY OF OBESITY

The World Health Organization have classified BMI as follows:

Classification	BMI (kg/m²)
Underweight	≤ 18.5
Healthy weight	18.5-24.9
Overweight	25-29.9
Obese	≥ 30

The BMI ranges are based on the effect body weight has on disease and death. As BMI increases, the risk for some disease increases. The BMI is the classification system used when discussing the prevalence of overweight and obesity within a population.

The BMI is used as a yardstick measure to classify individuals. However it doesn't take account of:

- Age
- Gender
- Fat distribution
- Weight associated with muscle and weight associated with fat.

Two people can have the same BMI, but a different per cent body fat. A bodybuilder with a large muscle mass and a low per cent body fat may have the same BMI as a person who has more body fat because BMI is calculated using weight and height only.

2. Waist circumference

Research has shown that excess fat stored in the abdominal area (around the belly) poses a higher risk to health than fat distributed elsewhere i.e. across the thighs and buttocks.

There are now guidelines to help identify those at increased risk due to their level of central obesity:

Increased Risk	
Men	≥ 94 cm (37")
Women	≥ 80cm (32")
Substantial Risk	
Men	≥ 102cm (40")
Women	≥ 88cm (35")

Obesity in the UK

In England, the prevalence of obesity has increased steadily during the last 50 years and since the 1980s the proportion of obese people has trebled. Currently, over 60% of the adult population are overweight (BMI>25kg/m²) and 22% of men and 23% of women are obese

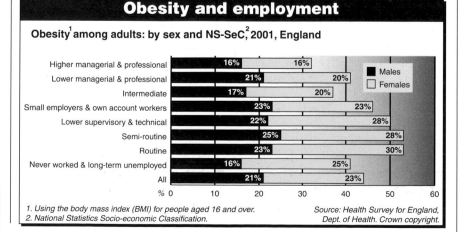

Obesity and employment

Obesity[1] among adults: by sex and NS-SeC,[2] 2001, England

	Males	Females
Higher managerial & professional	16%	16%
Lower managerial & professional	21%	20%
Intermediate	17%	20%
Small employers & own account workers	23%	23%
Lower supervisory & technical	22%	28%
Semi-routine	25%	28%
Routine	23%	30%
Never worked & long-term unemployed	16%	25%
All	21%	23%

1. Using the body mass index (BMI) for people aged 16 and over.
2. National Statistics Socio-economic Classification.

Source: Health Survey for England, Dept. of Health. Crown copyright.

(BMI>30kg/m^2). The prevalence of serious obesity increases with age. In 16- to 24-year-olds the prevalence is around 9% in men and 13% in women. By age 65-74 years the prevalence is over 28% in men and 30% in women; a three- to fourfold increase (HSE, 2003).

Historically, obesity was associated with affluence and this is still the case across societies. Within developing countries such as India, Africa and South America obesity is a particular problem amongst the recently affluent classes, where being overweight is seen as a sign of prosperity. However, in developed countries there is an inverse relationship between obesity and social class, with a much greater proportion of obese people in the lower social classes than in professional groups. In the UK the prevalence of serious obesity in women increases from 15.6% in social class I to 27.6% in social class V (HSE, 2003). Although a similar trend is observed in men, the social divide is not as significant (20.2% vs 21.0%).

Obesity in children

Less data are available about the prevalence of obesity in children. Moreover, due to difficulties in the definitions of overweight and obesity it is harder to make international comparisons (see ORIC backgrounder on Childhood Obesity). Figures from the Health Survey for England 2002 suggest one in 20 boys (5.5%) and about one in 15 girls (7.2%) aged 2-15 were obese. If figures for overweight are also

considered this increases the numbers of children at a weight that poses a risk to their health to 1 in 5 boys (21.5%) and 1 in 4 girls (27.5%). In 2001 in Scotland 10% of primary school entrants and 20% of primary school leavers [age 11/12] were obese. It is interesting to note that the Health Survey for England report describes the highest prevalence of childhood obesity in the most deprived areas of the UK, reflecting the trend observed in adults.

What can be done?

Although obesity is a rapidly growing problem there are some signs that it is not irreversible. In some western European countries, e.g. the Netherlands and some parts of Scandinavia, the prevalence of obesity is far lower than that seen in the UK and is increasing much more slowly.

In the UK there are many local initiatives under way to prevent and treat obesity, however there is currently no national strategy. Clinical guidelines for the treatment of obesity are available (cf. RCP and SIGN) and NICE has guidelines for the use of pharmacotherapy and surgery. Currently NICE is working on a more comprehensive series of clinical guidelines for prevention and treatment. Some other counties have made national plans to tackle the growing problem of obesity, for example 'Healthy Weight Australia'. Within many countries national Associations for the Study of Obesity bring together scientists and health professionals with an interest in obesity.

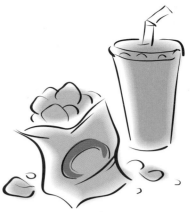

The Association for the Study of Obesity seeks to raise the awareness of obesity as a public health issue within the UK and to encourage research, and provides expert professional advice to Government and other organisations concerned with obesity issues.

On a global level, the International Obesity Task Force (IOTF) has been formed under the auspices of the International Association for the Study of Obesity (IASO). The IOTF includes obesity specialists from around the world. The main aims of the IOTF are:

The numbers of children at a weight that poses a risk to their health is 1 in 5 boys (21.5%) and 1 in 4 girls (27.5%)

- To raise awareness at all levels that obesity is a serious medical condition and a major global health problem.
- To develop policy recommendations for a coherent and effective global approach to manage and prevent obesity.
- To identify and implement strategies in collaboration with experts, professional organisations, patient groups and national health agencies.

The IOTF website can be found at: www.iotf.org

- Information reprinted with kind permission from the Association for the Study of Obesity. Visit www.aso.org.uk for more information or see page 41 for their contact details.

© ASO

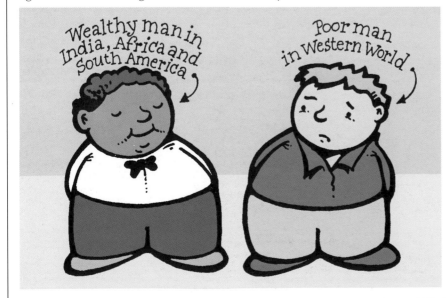

Wealthy man in India, Africa and South America

Poor man in Western World

Half of Britain fed up with healthy eating do-gooders!

Information from Mintel

A major new report from Mintel, looking at the nation's attitudes towards food, shows that half (48%) of all British adults are 'fed up with being told what to eat by "do-gooders" on healthy eating campaigns'. It would seem that a very sizeable portion of the British public is showing signs of health education 'overload', however well-intentioned the initiatives are.

Those aged 55-64 years old are the most likely to see themselves as being 'slightly overweight', which is consistent with more sedentary lifestyles

---

What is more, Mintel's exclusive consumer research reveals that many adults express an element of confusion over what actually constitutes healthy food. Around seven in 10 (69%) adults say 'it is hard to know which foods are healthy as advice from experts keeps changing', while almost three in five (58%) say that 'it is difficult to work out if foods are healthy from the labels or information on the pack'.

'There is clearly a large number of adults who are suffering from chronic information overload when it comes to healthy eating issues. Today, there is a wealth of information, which bombards the public in matters of health and diet, and given the complexity of many of these issues, it is hardly surprising that so many consumers feel confused. It seems they may now be in "switch off mode" when it comes to this advice, which has been named by Mintel as "do-gooder fatigue". Clearly, health education campaigners need to find new ways to encourage change for

MINTEL

the better in diet among this section of the population,' explains James McCoy, Senior Market Analyst at Mintel.

'That said, British eating habits remain sharply polarised, and at the other end of the spectrum Mintel anticipates the emergence of a so-called "Super Consumer". These forward-thinking Britons will take everything on board in terms of diet and health issues and will be more discerning about the food they put on their plate, be it for themselves, their partners or their family as a whole,' adds James McCoy.

Fat nation

Despite widespread irritation with healthy eating campaigns, the research also shows that around half of adults consider themselves to be overweight to some degree. In fact, some one in five (22%) feel that they are 'quite a bit overweight', with women (25%) more likely than men (18%) to feel this way.

'It is interesting to speculate whether there is any correlation between a relatively buoyant mood in the economy and spiralling levels of overweight and obese adults in Britain. It should be borne in mind, however, that eating habits tend to evolve over time, and that economic prosperity is likely to be only one aspect of a more complex set of factors behind the current so-called obesity epidemic,' adds James McCoy.

Those aged 55-64 years old are the most likely to see themselves as being 'slightly overweight', which is consistent with more sedentary lifestyles and a tendency to be fighting the classic middle-age spread. Interestingly, the 15- to 24-year-olds are the most likely to feel that they are 'about the right weight'.

What is naughty but nice when it comes to food?

Mintel's research shows that chocolate confectionery (31%) and crisps/bagged snacks (30%), both of which are heavily advertised, are the 'usual suspects' in terms of people's food weaknesses when it comes to weight. But Britain is clearly a nation of 'sweet tooths'. Indeed, some three out of the top four products people

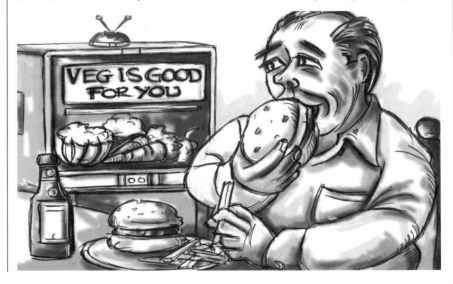

see as their weaknesses are sweet – chocolate bars, cakes and biscuits.

Somewhat surprisingly perhaps, wine (20%) is more likely to be seen as a weight weakness than beer (16%). These findings show just how popular wine has become in Britain over the last two decades, although more people still drink beer and lager than wine.

Overall in 2004, some 44% of women claimed to be trying to slim, compared to just 25% of men

---

It would seem that Atkins may also have had an effect on what people see as their food weaknesses. Some one in six (16%) adults see bread as their weakness, despite the Balance of Good Health model actually advocating eating more carbohydrates. This suggests that there is likely to be an 'Atkins effect', where carbohydrates are somewhat frowned upon as 'bad' foods, even if this is at odds with official health information advice.

Saturated with fat

Overall in 2004, some 44% of women claimed to be trying to slim, compared to just 25% of men. When it comes to cutting down on unhealthy food, the top three relate to cutting down the consumption of fat. Some two in five (39%) are at present or have in the past cut back on the amount of saturated fat they eat, making this the most popular change in eating habits. This is closely followed by switching to lower fat alternatives such as skimmed milk (34%), and eating fewer cooked breakfasts or grilling instead of frying (33%), both of which may simply be seen as fairly achievable healthy changes to make.

But it would seem that the British public are less stringent in efforts to curb their sweet tooth, as only a third (32%) of adults are cutting down on sugar and chocolate at present, or have done so in the past.

'This is a fairly modest response when considering the number of people who see sweet products as their weakness. This suggests that Britain is a nation of "sweet tooths", with many seeing a cutback on sweet treats such as chocolate bars as too much of a sacrifice. The fact is that foods such as chocolate are also important "mood foods", which for many satisfy an "emotional" need

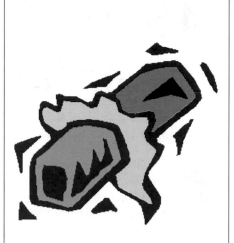

when bored or fed up. Indeed, some one in five (21%) adults snack because they are bored and a further one in ten (8%) snack when they are depressed,' explains James McCoy.

What is more, just one in five (21%) adults mention cutting down on crisps/nuts/snacks, once again falling short of the proportion who consider these products as the bane of their weight (30%). Findings again show the very 'moreishness' of bagged snacks and crisps in general.

Many adults are also not biting the bullet on their alcohol consumption. In fact, fewer than one in five (17%) adults either have or are currently cutting down the amount of alcohol they drink. Clearly drinking alcoholic beverages has become embedded in British cultural and recreational life.

About Mintel

Mintel is a worldwide leader of competitive media, product and consumer intelligence. For more than 30 years, Mintel has provided key insight into leading global trends. With offices in Chicago, London, Belfast and Sydney, Mintel's innovative product line provides unique data that have a direct impact on client success. For more information on Mintel, please visit their website at www.mintel.com.

■ The above information is reprinted with kind permission from Mintel – please visit their website at www.mintel.com for more information.

© Mintel

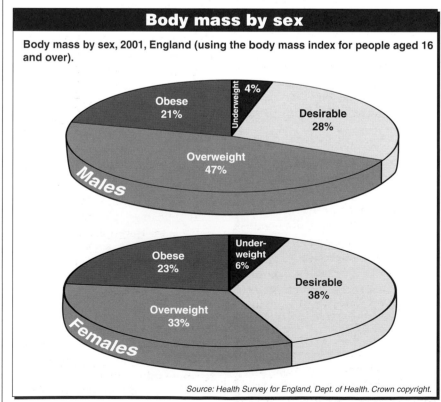

Body mass by sex

Body mass by sex, 2001, England (using the body mass index for people aged 16 and over).

Males
- Obese 21%
- Underweight 4%
- Desirable 28%
- Overweight 47%

Females
- Obese 23%
- Underweight 6%
- Desirable 38%
- Overweight 33%

Source: Health Survey for England, Dept. of Health. Crown copyright.

48 million adults unaware of health time bomb

'Measure your waist, measure your risk,' urges the National Obesity Forum

The majority of UK adults are unaware that having a large waist (abdominal obesity) is a root cause of diabetes and heart disease, according to a new survey. To highlight this, the National Obesity Forum (NOF), the UK's leading charity in the fight against obesity, today launched National Measure Your Waist Week, which calls us all to measure our waists.

The global survey reveals that 80% of those asked were unaware that abdominal obesity, which can be easily be detected by a simple tape measure round our waists, is linked to an increased risk of diabetes. And over 40% don't know that a fat tummy increases the risk of heart disease. Even more worryingly, the research also shows that although 77% of GPs are aware of abdominal obesity as a risk factor for type 2 diabetes and heart disease, only 18% of patients at risk of either type 2 diabetes or heart disease say their doctor has measured their waist.

'We are facing a public health time bomb and can't afford to be complacent about waist size,' said Dr Ian Campbell, GP and President of the NOF. 'We want National Measure Your Waist Week activity to raise awareness and encourage us all to measure our waists and seek medical advice if we're concerned at the size.'

The NOF will also be targeting Members of Parliament as they prepare to wine and dine during this year's party conference season. 'Our working hours and lifestyle are such that we MPs are notoriously bad at being able to keep to a healthy regime,' explained Dr Howard Stoate, Chair of the All Party Parliamentary Group on Obesity and member of the Health Select Committee, who is also a practising GP in his Dartford constituency. 'We do need to provide a lead in this area, though. If we don't then the current Government emphasis on individual responsibility will be hard to justify.'

Dr Campbell added: 'We want to encourage ministers to take action by pushing abdominal obesity higher up the healthcare agenda. Measuring waist circumference is a simple way to help identify patients at higher risk of heart disease and diabetes, yet, as the survey shows, waist size gets overlooked by many of my fellow colleagues.'

Recent studies suggest that using a tape measure could be a more accurate way of measuring your cardiovascular and metabolic risk than relying on body mass index (BMI) alone, which can be partic-

How to measure waist circumference

Waist circumference is a very different measurement to belt size. In order to accurately measure for abdominal fat, a major risk factor for heart disease and diabetes, it's important to measure the right part of your waist.

You can find out your waist circumference by following these four simple steps:
- Take off your shirt and loosen your belt.
- Place a tape measure around the waist at a point 1cm below the tummy button.
- Measure the waist circumference while breathing out, with the abdomen relaxed.
- Record the measurement. If you find you have a large waist measurement, speak to your healthcare professional to ask them what you could do to help decrease your waist circumference and your risk of diabetes and heart disease.

One-third of all Brits will be abdominally obese by the end of the next decade

ularly misleading if you are fit and carry a lot of muscle. According to leading guidelines, a waist circumference of more than 88 cm (35 inches) in women and 102 cm (40 inches) in men indicates the greatest risk for cardiovascular and metabolic disease. Additional guidelines indicate an increased risk at over 80cm and 94cm for women and men respectively.

Abdominal fat is now regarded as a root cause for developing cardiovascular abnormalities as well as metabolic complications such as abnormal cholesterol levels, insulin resistance and type 2 diabetes. It is calculated that the obesity-related illnesses, such as CVD, hypertension and type 2 diabetes, cost the NHS £386 million per year.

One-third of all Brits will be abdominally obese by the end of the next decade. Abdominal obesity, as measured by waist circumference, is one of the most common causes of heart disease and type 2 diabetes. Heart disease is Britain's biggest killer and diabetes, which can lead to life-threatening complications, affects over 1.8 million people in the UK.

More information on activities and the risks associated with abdominal obesity can be found at nationalmeasureyourwaistweek.org or by contacting the National Obesity Forum at their website: www.nationalobesityforum.org
19 September 2005

- Information from the National Obesity Forum. See page 41 or visit www.nationalobesityforum.org.uk for more information.

© National Obesity Forum

Being overweight is good for your health, says study

Being a little overweight is good for you, a study suggests. But being stick-thin – like some celebrities and supermodels – increases the risk of death, according to the research.

Overweight people are eating more healthily, exercising more, and controlling their blood pressure and cholesterol better than they used to

The startling findings are the result of a 'highly sophisticated' analysis by the American government watchdog, the Centres for Disease Control. Considered the most comprehensive ever undertaken, it agrees with several smaller studies in recent months. All show that those who are a little overweight have a lower risk of death than those of a normal weight.

As a result, US government experts have dramatically cut the annual number of deaths they blame on people being overweight – from 365,000 to just 25,814.

It means that, officially, more people – 34,000 – now die each year in the US because they are underweight rather than overweight. Most of these are aged 70 or older. The experts say the definition of a desirable weight range is probably now too low.

They emphasise, however, that there is a difference between being overweight, and being obese – obesity is still a major killer.

Researcher Dr David Williamson, who is overweight himself, said: 'If I had a family history – a father who had a heart attack at 52, or a brother

By Barry Wigmore

with diabetes – I would actively lose weight. As it is, I'm comfortable with my size.' The experts have changed their views on fat and thin people because the new study used more recent data and better statistical techniques, including factors such as smoking, age, race and alcohol consumption.

Based on the new calculations, excess weight drops from the second leading cause of preventable death – after smoking – to seventh.

Biostatistician Mary Grace Kovar said the classification for normal weight is now probably set too low. In addition, 'overweight' people are eating more healthily, exercising more, and controlling their blood pressure and cholesterol better than they used to.

She said: 'The researchers in this study have been very careful and are not overstating their case.'

Senior statistician Katherine Flegal, who led the study, said it raises questions on defining obesity.

The current method calculates BMI, or body-mass index, a person's weight-to-height ratio. It has been criticised for labelling superfit athletes obese because muscle weighs more than fat.
21 April 2005

© 2005 Associated Newspapers Ltd

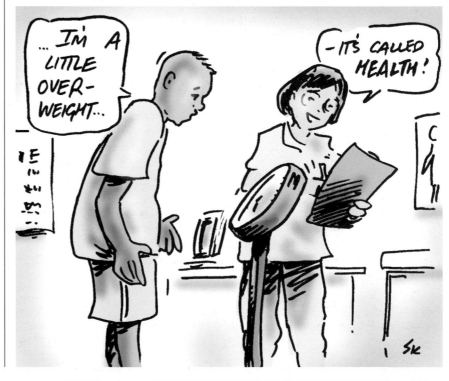

The question

Should employers avoid fat people?

By Tim Dowling

It's estimated that, in England and Wales, 18m working days a year are lost to obesity. Some studies also show that employees with a high body mass index (BMI) are less productive and more prone to absenteeism. Productivity and presenteeism aren't everything, of course, but Britain's employers are certainly put off by fat: a new poll of 2,000 personnel officers reveals that half of them believe overweight people lack self-discipline, and that obesity affects productivity. A third think that obesity is a valid medical reason for not hiring someone.

In America, where they're ahead of us on every level of this debate, Wal-Mart is trying, it was reported yesterday (27 October 2005), to incorporate physical exercise into every employee's job description, not to help the overweight get in shape, but to stop them applying for jobs in the first place – in their own words, 'to dissuade unhealthy people from coming to work at Wal-Mart' – thereby saving them an estimated $1bn a year in benefits.

Wal-Mart has never set much of an example in employee relations but their policy has implications for UK companies. Refusing to hire a specific fat person would be discriminatory, but there are no anti-fattist laws in the UK. The obese person's best hope of legal protection is the Disability Discrimination Act, though they would have to be fat enough to be considered disabled, or their fatness would have to be the cause of another disability – arthritis, perhaps – for them to make a case.

> *Britain's employers are certainly put off by fat: a new poll of 2,000 personnel officers reveals that half of them believe overweight people lack self-discipline, and that obesity affects productivity*

In the US, organisations such as the National Association to Advance Fat Acceptance (Naafa) have long championed the rights of the overweight. There, the debate has moved on to whether operations like stomach stapling should be covered by an employer's health plan (Wal-Mart – you guessed it – says no). This in turn has prompted a larger question: whether it's a surfeit of fatness or a simple dearth of fitness that is responsible for the sharp rise in employee ill-health. Is fatness an illness in itself, or just an impossible-to-conceal manifestation of health problems that bedevil the population as a whole? And, when everyone in America is overweight, who will do the discriminating?

28 October 2005

© *Guardian Newspapers Limited 2005*

Being overweight can impede job prospects

Information from Surgery Door

It is harder to find a job if you are overweight than if you are slim according to a survey of personnel officers.

According to the *Personnel Today* magazine survey of 2,000 people, most employers preferred to hire someone of 'normal' weight.

Half of the sample said they believed obesity affected a worker's productivity and a similar number thought overweight people lacked self-discipline.

One in 10 would not want an overweight employee to meet a client and the same percentage believed they could sack a worker for being fat, suggesting 'hidden' discrimination.

Karen Dempsey, editor of *Personnel Today*, said: 'To date, obesity has not been given the same recognition as sex, age, disabilities and race discrimination.

'But as our survey shows, overweight workers are being marginalised and given fewer opportunities than their slimmer counterparts.

'A clearer definition of obesity is needed to help businesses understand how obesity truly affects performance in the workplace.'

26 October 2005

■ The above information is reprinted with kind permission from Surgery Door. Visit www.surgerydoor.co.uk for more information.

© *Surgery Door*

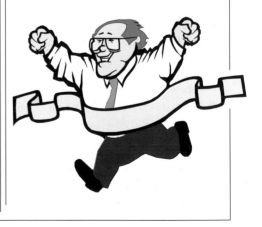

Snacking at work blamed for unfit employees

Information from *The Scotsman*

By *Louise Gray*

Snacking on unhealthy foods at work is not only making Scots fat but reducing productivity, a survey has found.

Almost three-quarters of Scots blamed a poor diet at work for weight gain and the same amount admitted the type of food they eat directly affects how well they work. The results have led doctors to call for a 'Jamie Oliver-style revolution' of the work canteen, with fruit replacing fry-ups.

> **Almost three-quarters of Scots blamed a poor diet at work for weight gain and the same amount admitted the type of food they eat directly affects how well they work**

The poll of more than 100 Scots was carried out by the health charity Developing Patient Partnerships (DPP) which is now launching a campaign to improve work eating and exercise habits: Working Your Way to a Fitter Day.

Workers said that stress and a lack of time leave little room for healthy eating. More than half admitted struggling with low energy levels as a result, with a quarter calling for afternoon naps to be allowed.

Yesterday (25 October 2005), a survey of 2,000 personnel officers found most believed obesity affected a worker's productivity and a similar number thought overweight people lacked self-discipline.

But Alison McGrory, a senior workplace promotion officer for Scotland's Health at Work, a body that provides free advice for companies on health, said improving health at work was not about criticising people for their weight but promoting a healthier lifestyle for all.

'It is not about pointing the finger and saying you are unhealthy because you are lazy, it is about helping people to make healthy choices,' she said.

Ms McGrory said people spend a large proportion of their time in work, so it was essential they eat well.

'Workplaces can do something tangible, rather than say "our workplace is really unhealthy because people have a poor diet" It is about thinking what workplaces can do to help people make that healthy choice.'

Dr Ian Campbell, the president of the National Obesity Forum, said healthy eating was essential for the economy.

'Jamie Oliver has highlighted the positive effects that healthy eating has on children during their day at school – we now need to ensure that this principle is applied to the workplace,' he said. 'Employers have enormous potential to gain from creating an environment which helps workers achieve healthier lifestyles and make healthy choices.'

Andrew Thomson, a GP in Tayside, said it was particularly important to introduce change in Scotland, where pie and chips is a staple of many canteens.

'As most people spend the majority of their week at work, it makes sense that information on how to incorporate healthy changes into their lives should be available at work, particularly as Scots have a reputation for poor diet and for generally unhealthy lifestyles,' he said.

Carina Norris, an Edinburgh nutritionist, said it is often difficult to find healthy alternatives.

'If there is a smart Edinburgh deli then you are lucky, but if the only place near your work is a burger bar it is more difficult,' she said.

'I am a firm believer in taking lunch to work if the alternative is fast food,' she added.

26 Ocotber 2005

© The Scotsman 2005

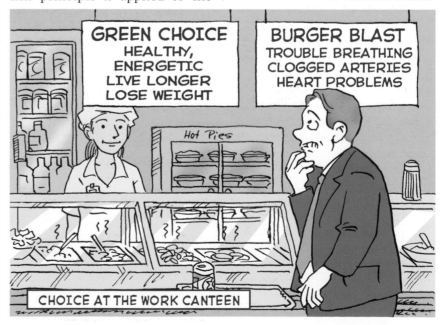

Facts about coronary heart disease

Information from the National Heart Forum

This article offers key facts and figures about the scale of the human, social and economic toll caused by coronary heart disease.

These are drawn largely from a detailed statistics database compiled and maintained by the British Heart Foundation.

Coronary heart disease is the leading single cause of death. It claimed the lives of over 125,000 people in the UK in 2000. One in four men and one in six women die from the disease

---

The database can be found at www.heartstats.org or via the BHF website. References are given below for information taken from sources other than the database.

Our research page gives information about current research in the field of coronary heart disease.

Total deaths from coronary heart disease

Coronary heart disease is the leading single cause of death. It claimed the lives of over 125,000 people in the UK in 2000. One in four men and one in six women die from the disease.

Coronary heart disease by itself is the most common cause of death in Europe: accounting for nearly two million deaths in Europe each year. Over one in five women (22%) and men (21%) die from the disease. In the European Union, coronary heart disease is also the most common single cause of death, with over 600,000 deaths every year.

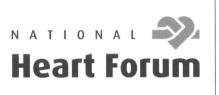

Premature deaths

Over 44,000 people under the age of 75 died from coronary heart disease in 2000. This represented 24% of all premature deaths among men and 14% of premature deaths among women.

Morbidity (illness and disability) caused by coronary heart disease

It is estimated that around 274,000 people have a heart attack each year in the UK and that about 2.1 million people have or have had angina (chest pain). The evidence is that although mortality from coronary heart disease is falling, morbidity is not falling and, in older age groups, is rising.

Social inequalities

Although death rates from coronary heart disease have fallen since the 1970s, the reductions have been greater among higher socio-economic groups. In England and Wales the premature death rate for male manual workers is 58% higher than for male non-manual workers. For women the rate is more than twice as high for manual compared with non-manual workers.

It is estimated that each year 5,000 lives and 47,000 working years are lost in men aged 20-64 years due to social class inequalities in coronary heart disease death rates (England and Wales).

Smoking

It is estimated that about 20% of deaths from coronary heart disease in men and 17% in women are due to smoking.

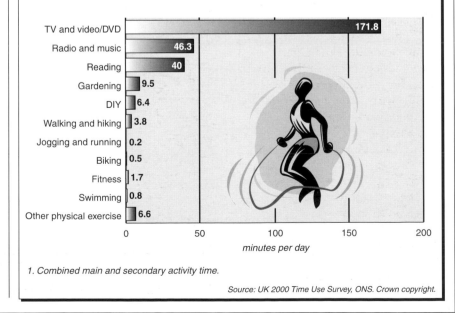

Time use and exercise

Average time spent on various activities,[1] United Kingdom, 2000.

Activity	minutes per day
TV and video/DVD	171.8
Radio and music	46.3
Reading	40
Gardening	9.5
DIY	6.4
Walking and hiking	3.8
Jogging and running	0.2
Biking	0.5
Fitness	1.7
Swimming	0.8
Other physical exercise	6.6

1. Combined main and secondary activity time.

Source: UK 2000 Time Use Survey, ONS. Crown copyright.

One in two long-term smokers will die prematurely of smoking-related diseases – half of these in middle age.[1]

Diet

It is estimated that up to 30% of deaths from coronary heart disease are due to unhealthy diets.

Only a small proportion of adults and children eat the recommended daily intake of five portions of fruit and vegetables.[2] Adults eat on average around three portions a day (with lower rates among low-income groups). Children eat on average only about two portions a day. Consumption of fruit and vegetables in the UK is about half that of Greece, Italy and Spain.[3]

The percentage of food energy derived from total fat in the British diet is falling only gradually. From 42% in the mid-1970s it has fallen to just under 39%. The percentage of food energy derived from saturated fat has fallen more dramatically – from around 20% to about 15% – but still exceeds the COMA recommendation of not more than 10% of food energy.[4]

Physical acitvity

It is estimated that about 36% of deaths from coronary heart disease in men and 38% of deaths in women are due to lack of physical activity.

It is estimated that 9% of deaths from coronary heart disease in the UK could be avoided if people who are currently sedentary or have a light level of physical activity increased it to a moderate level.

Levels of physical activity in the UK are below the European Union average.

Overweight and obesity

Inactivity, together with a poor diet, is leading to rising rates of overweight and obesity, increasing the risk of chronic diseases in later life, including coronary heart disease and diabetes. The prevalence of high blood pressure and diabetes is three times higher among overweight people than among those of normal body weight, and obesity is also associated with higher levels of total blood cholesterol.[5]

Inactivity, together with a poor diet, is leading to rising rates of overweight and obesity, increasing the risk of chronic diseases in later life, including coronary heart disease and diabetes

---

The number of obese six-year-olds doubled in the last ten years and the number of obese 15-year-olds more than trebled. Between 1980 and 1997 the prevalence of overweight adults in England increased from 39% to 62% of men, and from 32% to 53% of women, and the percentage of these who are clinically obese rose from 6% to 17% in men, and from 8% to 20% in women.

Economic costs

Coronary heart disease cost the UK healthcare system about £1,600 million in 1996. The cost of hospital care for people with the disease accounted for 54% of these costs. Thirty-two per cent was accounted for by the cost of drugs and dispensing them. Only 1% of such costs was spent on the prevention of coronary heart disease.

References

1   Scientific Committee on Tobacco and Health, 1998.
2   Department of Health, 2000. *National Diet and Nutrition Survey: Young people aged 4 to 18 years. Volume 1. Report of the Diet and Nutrition Survey.* London: The Stationery Office.
3   Food and Agriculture Organization Agrostat Supply Data, 1992.
4   Committee on Medical Aspects of Food Policy, 1994. *Nutritional aspects of cardio-vascular disease: Report of the Cardiovascular Review Group. Report on health and social subjects number 46.* London: The Stationery Office.
5   Brownson RC, Remington PL, Davis JR, for the American Public Health Association. 1993. *Chronic disease epidemiology and control.* Baltimore (USA): Port City Press.

■ Information reprinted with kind permission from the National Heart Forum. Visit www.heartforum.org.uk for more information or if you wish to write to them, please see page 41 for contact details.

© *National Heart Forum*

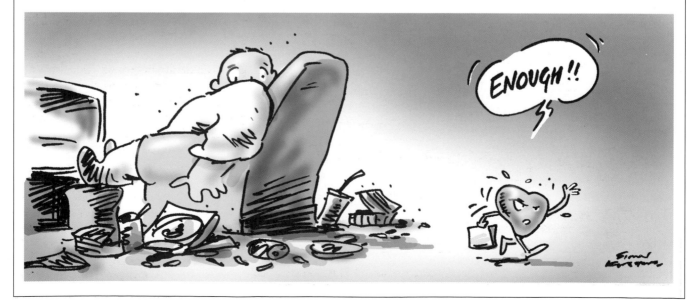

Get active!

Information from the British Heart Foundation

What does it mean to be more active?

Being physically active might involve going swimming, doing an exercise class or playing a sport, but it also includes everyday things such as walking, gardening and climbing stairs. You can get the benefits of being more active from all types of physical activity, not just from formal 'exercise'.

Why should I be more active?

Being active will make a difference to your quality of life. Once you start, the benefits will become obvious. You'll experience:

- Better health
- More energy – you'll be able to cope with your daily routine and have energy to spare
- Reduced stress – you'll relax more easily and feel better about yourself

- Stronger bones and muscles
- Better balance, strength, suppleness and mobility
- More independence in later life – you'll be able to cope with daily tasks more easily
- Improved sleep
- Better maintenance of a healthy weight
- More social opportunities – you'll meet other people who enjoy being active
- A sense of achievement
- Increased enjoyment – activity can be fun and it's something you could do as a family.

Physical activity improves both your physical and mental health. It is one of the most important factors in maintaining a good quality of life. The heart is a muscle, but it's the most important muscle we've got, and it needs exercise to keep fit so that it can pump blood efficiently with each heart beat.

If you are already regularly active, you can still benefit by adding more activity. Generally, the more active you are, the more benefits you will get.

Who can benefit from being more active?

Everyone can benefit – whatever your age, size or physical condition. Just remember that you are never too old or too unfit to start doing something. In fact, the greatest increase in health benefit comes to inactive people who start to take regular moderate physical activity. Your health risks will decrease as soon as you start to do more.

How much do you do already?

How many days of the week do you do something active? (Think about activities both at work and in your leisure time.) When you are physically active, how much time do you put into it? (Add up all the minutes from all activities.) Read on to find out just how much you need to do to ensure health benefits and improve the quality of your life.

How much activity should I be doing?

Any increase in activity will benefit your health but experts agree that all adults should aim to build up to at least 30 minutes of moderate intensity physical activity on 5 or more days of the week.

Your health risks will decrease as soon as you start to do more.

- The above information is taken from the document *Get Active!* from the British Heart Foundation. Visit www.bhf.org.uk to view the full document or see page 41 for details.

© *British Heart Foundation*

Exercise and health

Health problem	How activity can help
Coronary heart disease and stroke	Inactivity is one of the major causes of coronary heart disease and stroke in Britain. People who are inactive have twice the risk of developing coronary heart disease compared with active people. Regular activity slows down the narrowing of the arteries to the heart and brain that occurs with age. The more exercise you do, the stronger and more efficient the heart becomes so it can pump more blood with each beat.
High blood pressure	Physical activity can help to reduce high blood pressure. It also reduces the likelihood of developing it in the first place. If you have high blood pressure, avoid certain 'weight-boaring' acitivities such as lifting weights in a gym
Stress, anxiety and depression	Being active has been shown to help with each of these. It is a great means of letting off steam and will leave you feeling revitalised and relaxed.
Overweight and obesity	Regular physical activity is crucial to preventing obesity and in helping people to lose weight. Activity encourages the body to use up excess stored fat. Remember that losing weight involves both eating healthily and increasing the amount of exercise you do.
Type 2 diabetes	Activity helps you maintain normal blood glucose levels. Regular activity helps in the prevention and management of diabetes.
Osteoporosis (thinning of the bones)	Most physical acitvities improve balance and muscle strength, which reduces the risk of falling. Any weight-bearing acitivity (such as stair-climbing and walking) will strengthen bones and reduce the risk of fracture.
Certain cancers	Some forms of cancer are less likely to occur in people who are physically active.
Abnormal blood cholesterol levels	Cholesterol is a fatty substance mainly made in the body by the liver. Physical activity helps to improve your cholesterol levels by increasing the level of more protective high density lipoprotein (HDL) in the blood.

Source: 'Get Active!', © the British Heart Foundation.

Why exercise is wise

Information from KidsHealth

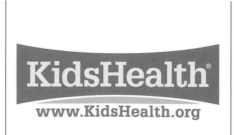

You've probably heard countless times how exercise is 'good for you' but did you know that it can actually help you feel good, too? Getting the right amount of exercise can rev up your energy levels and even help you to feel better emotionally.

Experts recommend that adults get more than 60 minutes of moderate to vigorous physical activity each day. There are three components to a well-balanced exercise routine: aerobic exercise, strength training, and flexibility training.

Rewards and benefits

Exercise benefits every part of the body, including the mind. Exercising causes the body to produce endorphins, chemicals that lead a person to feel peaceful and happy. Exercise can help some people sleep better. It can also help with mental health issues such as mild depression and self-esteem: if you feel strong and powerful, it can help you see yourself in a better light. Plus, exercise can give people a real sense of accomplishment and pride at having achieved a certain goal – like beating an old time in the 100-metre dash.

Exercising can help you look better, too. People who exercise burn calories and look more toned than those who don't. In fact, exercise is one of the most important parts of keeping your body at a healthy weight. When you exercise, you burn food calories as fuel. If a person eats more calories than he or she burns, the body stores them away as fat. Exercise can help burn these stored calories.

Exercising to maintain a healthy weight also decreases a person's risk of developing certain diseases, including type 2 diabetes and high blood pressure. These diseases, which used to be found mostly in adults, are becoming more common in teens.

Finally, it may not seem important now, but exercise can help a person age well. Women are especially prone to a condition called osteoporosis (a weakening of the bones) as they get older. Studies have found that weight-bearing exercise, like running or brisk walking, can help girls (and guys!) keep their bones strong.

Aerobic exercise

Like other muscles, the heart likes a good workout. You can provide it with one in the form of aerobic exercise. Aerobic exercise is any type of exercise that gets the heart pumping and the muscles using oxygen (you'll notice your body using oxygen as you breathe faster). When you give your heart this kind of workout on a regular basis, your heart will get stronger and more efficient in delivering oxygen (in the form of oxygen-carrying blood cells) to all parts of your body.

Experts recommend that adults get more than 60 minutes of moderate to vigorous physical activity each day

In addition to being active every day, experts recommend that teens get at least three 20-minute sessions a week of vigorous activity. If you play team sports, you're probably doing more than that recommendation, which is great! Some team sports that give you a great aerobic workout are swimming, basketball, soccer, lacrosse, hockey, and rowing.

But if you don't play team sports, don't worry; there are plenty of ways to get aerobic exercise on your own or with friends. These include biking, running, swimming, dancing, in-line skating, cross-country skiing, hiking, and walking quickly. In fact, the types of exercise that you do on your own are easier to continue when you leave high school and go on to work or college, making it easier to stay fit later in life as well.

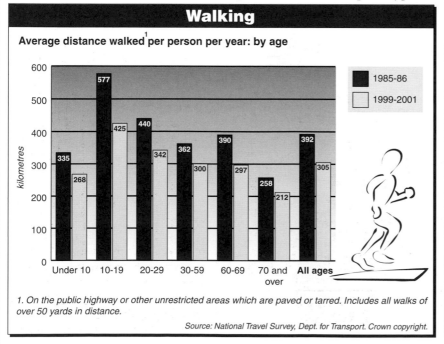

Walking

Average distance walked[1] per person per year: by age

Legend: ■ 1985-86 □ 1999-2001

Age	1985-86	1999-2001
Under 10	335	268
10-19	577	425
20-29	440	342
30-59	362	300
60-69	390	297
70 and over	258	212
All ages	392	305

(y-axis: kilometres)

1. On the public highway or other unrestricted areas which are paved or tarred. Includes all walks of over 50 yards in distance.

Source: National Travel Survey, Dept. for Transport. Crown copyright.

Strength training

The heart isn't the only muscle to benefit from regular exercise – most of the other muscles in your body enjoy exercise, too. When you use your muscles and they become stronger, it allows you to be active for longer periods of time without getting worn out. Strong muscles are also a plus because they actually help protect you when you exercise by supporting your joints and helping to prevent injuries. Muscle also burns more energy when a person's at rest than fat does, so building your muscles will help you burn more calories and maintain a healthy weight.

Muscle burns more energy when a person's at rest than fat does, so building your muscles will help you burn more calories and maintain a healthy weight

Different types of exercise strengthen different muscle groups, for example:

- For arms, try rowing or cross-country skiing. Pull-ups and push-ups, those old gym class standbys, are also good for building arm muscles.
- For strong legs, try running, biking, or skating.
- For shapely abs, you can't beat rowing, bike riding, and crunches.

Flexibility training

Strengthening the heart and other muscles isn't the only important goal of exercise. Exercise also helps the body stay flexible, meaning that your muscles and joints stretch and bend easily. People who are flexible can worry less about strained muscles and sprains. Flexibility can also help improve a person's sports performance. Some activities, like dance or martial arts, obviously require great flexibility, but increased flexibility can also help people perform better at other sports, such as soccer or lacrosse.

Sports and activities that encourage flexibility are easy to find. Many high schools have gymnastics programs. Martial arts like karate also help a person stay flexible. Ballet, pilates, and yoga are other good choices. Warming up for a workout and doing simple stretching exercises after your workout also help you develop flexibility.

What's right for me?

One of the biggest reasons people drop an exercise programme is lack of interest: if what you're doing isn't fun, it's hard to keep it up. The good news is that there are tons of different sports and activities that you can try out to see which one inspires you.

When picking the right type of exercise for you it can help to consider your workout personality. For example, do you like to work out alone and on your own schedule (in which case solo sports like biking or snowboarding may be for you), or do you like the shared motivation and companionship that comes from being part of a team? You also need to factor in practical considerations, such as whether your chosen activity is affordable and accessible to you (activities like horse riding are harder for people who live in cities, for example) and how much time you can set aside for your sport.

Too much of a good thing

Like all good things, it's possible to overdose on exercise. Although exercising is a great way to maintain

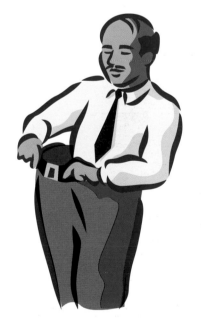

a healthy weight, exercising too much to lose weight isn't healthy. The body needs enough calories to function properly. Remember that you're still growing and will continue to do so throughout your teen years. You'll need the energy to fuel the growth.

Exercising too much in an effort to burn calories and lose weight can be a sign of an eating disorder. If you have any doubts about how much you should be exercising, talk with a school nurse or family doctor. And if you ever get the feeling that your exercise is in charge of you rather than the other way around, talk with your doctor, a parent, or another adult you trust.

Some girls who overexercise may stop getting their periods, a condition known as amenorrhoea (pronounced: a-meh-nuh-ree-uh). Girls who regularly miss periods are less able to incorporate calcium into their bones, which can lead to the decreased bone density and increased risk of injury that goes with osteoporosis. The combination of amenorrhoea, disordered eating, and osteoporosis is a condition called female athlete triad.

Considering the benefits to the heart, muscles, joints, and mind, it's easy to see why exercise is wise. If you exercise now, keep it up as you become an adult (this is often the biggest exercise challenge for people as they get busy with college and careers). One of the great things about exercise is that it's never too late to start. And don't forget that even small things can count as exercise when you're starting out – like taking a short bike ride or raking leaves. Even walking your dog counts as part of your 60 minutes a day of exercise (and your vet will tell you that animals need workouts just like humans do, so if your family pooch is portly, he'll benefit from your dedication, too).

- This information was provided by KidsHealth, one of the largest resources online for medically reviewed health information for parents, kids and teens. For more articles like this one, visit their websites at www.teenshealth.org or www.kidshealth.org

© 1995-2005. *The Nemours Foundation*

Getting fit

The smart guide to shaping up

What exactly does 'fit' mean?

Different authorities have differing opinions on what makes someone 'fit'. The bottom line is this: if you're physically fit, you can do your chosen form of exercise without ending up completely exhausted. To do this you need: strength, endurance, speed, flexibility, and so on (see our glossary at the bottom for more details). To be good at a particular sport (also called motor fitness), you might also need quick reaction times, agility, balance, co-ordination, and power.

Fit me up, then!

If you've decided to get fit, don't keep putting it off: procrastination is deadly. Then again, a little thought is needed first, rather than going at it hell for leather. People who go straight in without any knowledge or the right gear can earn some serious chafing and blisters, making them more likely to give up.

Most trainers suggest that you should start gradually and build up from there. If you're completely unfit or have had any illness or ongoing health problem, consult your doctor before starting an exercise regime. Exercise can improve many health conditions, but check first, in case you have something that needs temporary rest. Make sure you're wearing the right clothing and have the correct safety equipment if required.

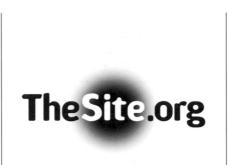

Pick a form of exercise that you can do frequently and will enjoy. You can also mix up the types of exercise that you do, for all-round body conditioning. Remember that getting fit can take several weeks or months. It's easy to get frustrated or give up, but hang in there. You should see some obvious results within six to eight weeks.

A simple plan

The first phase: get your body used to frequent moderate levels of activity for the first four to six weeks. Your exercise should include stretching and a warm-up, continuous aerobic activity, some toning exercises, and a warm-down afterwards. To see benefits you need to do enough to increase your heart rate (to between 60 and 70% of its maximum) and make you breathe deeper.

Improvers: increase your levels of activity slightly every couple of weeks. Your body is adapting to the exercise, so you need to push it slightly harder to keep getting results. Increase the length of your exercise sessions, or the intensity of them.

Maintenance: after about six months, the average person has reached a level of fitness that they're happy with, and decides to stick with their current level of exercise to maintain their fitness. If you're training for sport or competitions, you will probably need to push yourself for longer.

Fitness glossary

Agility: being able to go through a series of fast and powerful movements.

Balance: being able to control the position of the body either when moving or when still.

Cardio-respiratory endurance: how effective your heart and lungs are at getting oxygen and fuel around the body for movement, and how well your body uses them.

Co-ordination: being able to integrate agility and balance, to move effectively.

Flexibility: the range of movements that you have in your joints.

Muscular (or strength) endurance: how well your muscle fibres can repeatedly do the same actions without tiring. Sometimes called stamina.

Power: your ability to make fast and controlled muscular contractions, in an explosive burst.

Speed: your ability to move a set distance in a certain time.

Strength: the maximum force that your muscles can produce by contracting against resistance. Someone who is very strong may appear fit, but could have very little stamina or flexibility.

■ The above information is reprinted with kind permission from TheSite.org. Visit www.thesite.org for more information.

© TheSite.org

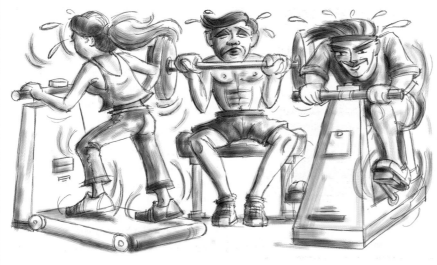

Physical activity

Information from BUPA

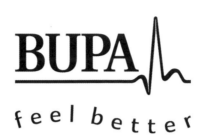

For thousands of years, physical activity has been associated with health. Today, science has confirmed the link, with over-whelming evidence that people who lead active lifestyles are less likely to die early, or to experience major illnesses such as heart disease, diabetes and colon cancer.

But it's often difficult to change exercise habits. Thinking about your motivation can help.

Exercise facts

Evidence shows that regular exercise can:

- increase levels of HDL or 'good' cholesterol,
- lower high blood pressure,
- help improve body composition by burning fat,
- promote healthy blood sugar levels,
- promote bone density,
- boost the immune system,
- improve mood and reduce the chance of depression.

Despite the strong case for staying active, many people find it difficult to adapt their daily lives to in-corporate physical activity. With cars on most driveways and the decline in the number of physically active jobs, 70% of the adult population is sufficiently inactive to be classed as 'sedentary'. Being sedentary increases the risk of a heart attack or stroke by the same amount as smoking.

In practice, it seems that the threat of a future illness is often not enough motivation for people to change their habits.

Barriers to being more active

People give many reasons for not taking up exercise:

- lack of time due to work or family commitments,
- cost of equipment or gym membership,
- lack of facilities nearby,
- personal safety when exercising outdoors alone,
- poor weather or night-time lighting.

However, there are ways to get round all of these potential barriers. For example, by getting off the bus to school or work one or two stops earlier than usual, which is free and requires no special equipment or facilities.

The moderate message

Many people are put off physical activity because they believe that only vigorous exercise or playing sport counts as healthy activity. But,

in fact, substantial health benefits can be achieved from regular activity without the need for special equipment, sporting ability or getting very hot and sweaty.

There is now strong scientific evidence that moderate intensity physical activity – equivalent to brisk walking for 30 minutes per day on most days of the week – is enough to bring about real benefits in terms of promoting health and preventing illnesses.

Despite the strong case for staying active, many people find it difficult to adapt their daily lives to incorporate physical activity

---

Regular activity can also improve the way you look and feel. In combination with a balanced diet, regular activity can help to maintain a healthy weight. It can even boost self-confidence and reduce the risk of depression.

How much is enough?

For an adult, regular, moderate intensity physical activity means using up about an extra 200 calories per day, most days of the week. This equates to about 30 minutes of activity, such as a two-mile brisk walk, that should make you feel warm and mildly out of breath. During moderate intensity activity, you should still be able to talk without panting in between your words.

If you have previously been inactive and 30 minutes of activity per day sounds like a tall order, the good news is that separate sessions of ten minutes can count towards the total.

It's possible to achieve your 30-minute target by making fairly simple changes to your everyday routine,

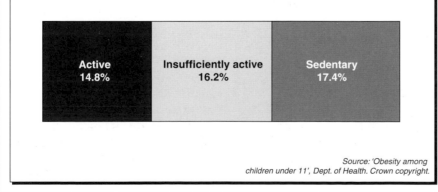

Child obesity and physical activity

Obesity prevalence among children aged 2-10 classified obese, by child physical activity status

| Active 14.8% | Insufficiently active 16.2% | Sedentary 17.4% |

Source: 'Obesity among children under 11', Dept. of Health. Crown copyright.

without joining the gym or running a marathon.

Examples of everyday activities that count:

- walking up stairs instead of using lifts,
- walking up moving escalators,
- for short journeys, walking instead of driving,
- doing the housework at 'double-time',
- DIY and gardening, such as painting or raking leaves.

Keeping fit

Your ability to keep up a physical activity such as jogging, racket sports, cycling or swimming, is related to your aerobic fitness – or stamina.

Generally speaking, the greater your stamina, the greater are the health benefits. If you want to improve your stamina, it's important to start gently, increasing the frequency of your activity before increasing how hard you exercise.

Staying motivated

Even when you usually enjoy exercising, there will be days when you just can't seem to find the motivation to get active. Here are some practical tips to help keep up enthusiasm:

- Keep a diary. Whatever sport or activity you do, this can help you. Note down how far you ran or the match score, your pulse, how you felt etc. That way you can look back and see how you have improved over time.
- Collect inspiration. Stick quotes from coaches, athletes, or anyone successful around your house and/ or your office. Inspirational stories from people who have achieved against the odds may help – if they can do it, so can you.

When it comes to staying motivated it's just as important to train your brain as it is to train your body. Here are just a few ideas to help you win the mental battle and stay on the exercise track.

- Set yourself some short and long-term goals. Success will provide you with a sense of satisfaction and further motivation to keep up the new lifestyle. Keep your goals SMART:

  Specific
  Measurable
  Achievable
  Realistic
  Time-based

  For example, rather than saying you'll get fit by summer, start by setting the more specific goal of going to an hour-long fitness class every week.
- A great way to stay focused is to keep reminding yourself of the reasons that motivated you to start exercising in the first place

Have fun

The key to keeping up with a resolution to get fit is finding an activity, or range of activities, that you enjoy. Not everyone sees exercise as fun, and doing something you find boring just because it's good for you is very difficult to sustain. But you can take steps to make it more enjoyable.

Try out new sports or activities until you find something you like. When you find an activity you like, try exercising with a friend, at a pace that still allows you to talk. Activities that you can do as a family or with friends may help with motivation.

Perhaps try actitivies to music, such as dance or aerobics, and make sure you vary your activity a little so you don't get bored. Try exercising in beautiful scenery, such as on a beach or in a park. Maybe you could buy yourself some new exercise clothes that you like wearing and feel good in.

e.g. the aim of losing weight, improving your health, or testing yourself in a competition by taking part in a race.

- Visualisation. Picture yourself achieving your goal, such as completing a race or slipping into the next size down in trousers, and imagine what it will feel like. These images and feelings will help to motivate you to achieving them for real.
- Enjoy it! Exercising releases chemicals in the brain, such as serotonin, that have a strong affect on your mood, helping reduce anxiety, stress and depression. So whenever you don't feel like exercising, try to remind yourself how good you'll feel afterwards.

- The above information is reprinted with kind permission from BUPA, excluding any accompanying illustrations, diagrams and graphs. Visit www.bupa.co.uk/health for more information or see page 41 for their address details.

© BUPA

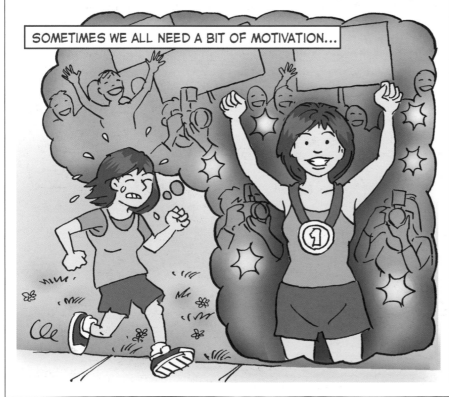

SOMETIMES WE ALL NEED A BIT OF MOTIVATION...

Physical exercise

The good news is you don't have to be good at sport to be active. Small changes to your everyday routine, such as walking or cycling to school, increase your activity and help you to feel and look good. Activities like dancing and roller-blading are also a great way of increasing your activity and having fun at the same time!

As well as having fun, taking part in physical activity is a great way to:
- reduce boredom
- meet up with your mates and also meet new people
- unwind from your studies and relieve stress and tension.

And there are also lots of benefits to your health:
- weight control
- helping you to breathe more easily, which is especially important if you have asthma
- building stronger bones.

How much should I do?

Most young people of school age are physically active for about half an hour a day, most days of the week. This may sound good, but it's not enough to get the full health benefit. Ideally, you should be aiming for one hour of moderate intensity activity each day.

Moderate intensity activity makes you feel warm and breathe more heavily than usual. More vigorous activity is fine as long as you feel okay and still able to talk. This is known as your comfort zone. If you are unable to do this, you are probably working at too high an intensity. Check out your comfort zone.

You don't have to do one hour of activity all in one go. You can build up over the day – for example, 10 minutes walking to school, 20 minutes basketball at lunchtime, 10 minutes walking home from school and 20 minutes dancing around your room to your favourite tunes! Every little bit counts, but try to include some activity that is non-stop for 10-15 minutes – this would really help your heart health.

Warming up

For moderate to vigorous activities, you need to prepare your body for action. Your warm-up can be changed for different activities, but should include:

Activities that gradually raise the pulse
- Start with some gentle activity to gradually increase your heart rate. This ensures that the body is prepared gradually for the demands being made on it. Activities may include walking, gentle jogging, or cycling in a low gear.

Activities to mobilise the joints
- Mobility exercises involve slow, controlled movements of the muscles around those joints that will be used in the activity. For example, shoulder rotations, side bends and knee lifts.
- These should be performed with control, avoiding rapid flinging actions. Stand in a comfortable position, with knees slightly bent and feet apart, and repeat each movement 6 to 8 times.

Stretching
- It is important to stretch the main muscle groups to be used in the activity for 6-10 seconds. For example, if the activity mainly involves leg work, stretches for the major leg muscles – the calves, quadriceps, hamstrings and groin – are required.

Cooling down

A cool-down after any moderate to vigorous physical activity will help to reduce the stiffness you sometimes get after activity. In the same way that the intensity of activity is gradually increased in the warm-up, it should be gradually decreased in the cool-down. The main types of activity that should be included are:

Activities to decrease the pulse rate
- One of the most effective cool-down activities is walking. Start with power walking, move through race walking and brisk walking and end with gentle walking.

Stretching
- A cool-down should include stretches for the muscle groups used in the activity. Stretches carried out in the warm-up can be repeated, but should be held for a minimum of 10-20 seconds and up to 60 seconds, where comfortable.

- The above information is from the government's mind, body and soul website which can be found at: www.mindbodysoul.gov.uk

© Crown copyright

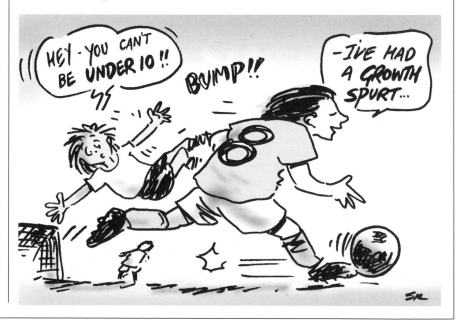

Student fitness

Moving into higher education introduces you to a whole new range of leisure opportunities that you might never have thought about before. It's a chance to try out all kinds of different activities, usually for free or at very low cost. So what have you got to lose? By Karla Fitzhugh

So many options

Most colleges have a gym, swimming pool or sports ground, and various classes and clubs to try out. If you are the sort of person who likes a bit of competition then you might have difficulty choosing between football, squash, basketball, rugby, netball, tennis, hockey, cricket, badminton, water polo, athletics and volleyball.

In the gym you can try your hand at ju jitsu, kickboxing, and akido, different kinds of aerobics, step workouts or body conditioning. If you want to tone up you can also try weight training, classes like 'Tums and Bums', boxercise, or circuit training.

Even if you don't think of yourself as the traditional sporty type, there are many other ways to get fit and stay healthy

Even if you don't think of yourself as the traditional sporty type, there are many other ways to get fit and stay healthy, including tai chi,

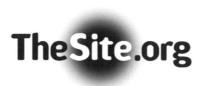

women's self defence, yoga and the martial arts. Those who crave more adventure can get their adrenaline fixes by going out rock climbing, orienteering, horse riding, scuba diving, hang gliding, potholing, skiing, canoeing, parachuting, hiking and hot air ballooning. If you haven't seen anything that takes your fancy yet then it's relatively easy to get a few people together and start a club of your own.

Why bother?

But why should anybody bother getting all hot and sweaty when they could be at home nice and comfy watching daytime television or out drinking subsidised lager in the union bar all night? The good news is that you only need to take two or three hours out of this thrilling weekly schedule to get all the benefits – and,

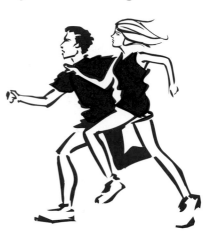

let's face it, reruns of Ironside and Columbo will have lost their sparkle long before the end of the first term, and it's only a matter of time before This Morning starts getting on your nerves too.

Boosting your fitness levels will give you more energy and help you sleep better. Feeling like you are getting into shape also gives you a confidence boost. Regular exercise is a great stress buster, which is good to remember at exam time, and can even help relieve the symptoms of mild depression. Looking even further ahead, it can make a useful contribution to a CV when you are looking for work after graduation, so it might even give you the edge in landing your dream job. Employers value skills like teamwork, self-discipline and coping well with responsibility.

Keeping fit is also an easy way to make new friends, and lots of clubs organise social outings and parties, or just meet up regularly for drinks. And, of course, a fit body is an attractive body – which might well be a factor in meeting that special someone . . .

■ The above information is from TheSite.org's website which can be found at www.thesite.org

© TheSite.org

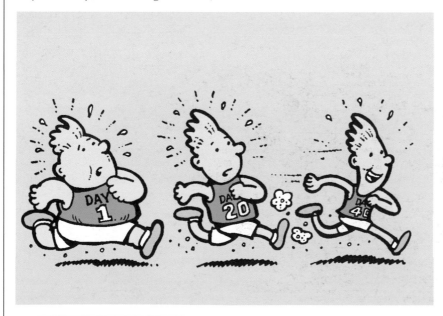

Exercise beats the blues

Information from BUPA

Exercise may be just as effective at treating depression as antidepressant medicines, according to a report from the Mental Health Foundation.

The report also claims that being physically active may help to prevent you from developing depression in the first place.

What does the report say?

The report says that several studies have shown exercise to be an effective treatment for depression. It also states that exercise therapy should be used as a first-line treatment for mild depression because it may be just as effective as antidepressant medicines.

The government advises that antidepressant medicines and psychological therapies should be offered when simpler methods (such as self-help or exercise) have failed to adequately treat the symptoms of mild depression.

What is depression?

Depression is a long-lasting low mood that interferes with your day-to-day life. It is very common, affecting about one in six people at some point in their lives. It is often triggered by a traumatic event.

What are the symptoms of depression?

In addition to feeling sad, some people with depression are irritable and may lose their temper more easily than usual. They tend to feel separate from everyone else and find that they can't enjoy events or activities that they normally would.

People with depression may also have:

- less energy than usual
- tiredness
- poor concentration
- difficulty sleeping (problems getting to sleep, waking up unrefreshed from a long sleep, or waking up very early)
- loss of sex drive

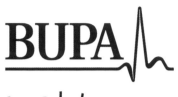

- disturbed eating patterns – either loss of appetite or eating too much (comfort eating).

For more information on depression, please see BUPA's Depression factsheet.

What causes depression?

Anyone can have depression and it can develop for no apparent reason. Some events may trigger depression, such as:

- bereavement
- relationship problems
- money worries
- stress at work
- fear of losing your job or being made redundant
- moving home
- long-term or serious illness (such as diabetes or cancer)

- having a baby (postnatal depression).

How is depression normally treated?

Depression is commonly treated using antidepressant medicines and talking therapies that look at different ways of thinking about and coping with problems. Doctors tend to favour psychotherapy and counselling for treating depression in its early stages. Unfortunately these are often in short supply and you may be asked to join a waiting list.

Exercise therapy should be used as a first-line treatment for mild depression

---

But exercise therapy may be just as effective for treating the early stages of depression. Regular exercise may also help protect people from becoming depressed in the first place.

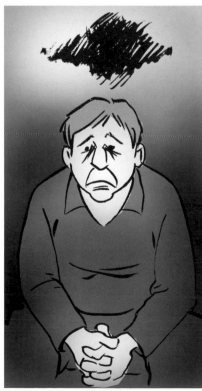

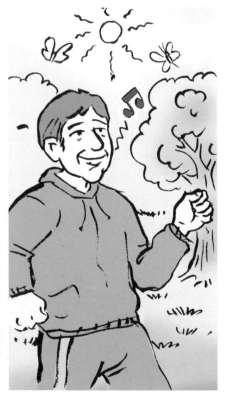

How might exercise help treat depression?

Exercise appears to help people feel better by:

- improving their mood
- reducing their anxiety
- improving concentration
- enhancing their view of themselves
- reducing stress
- improving sleep.

Why does exercise help lift depression?

No one knows exactly why exercise helps to relieve depression but it is likely to be due to a number of different reasons.

- Physical activity increases the amount of hormones (endorphins) in our bodies that help you to feel happy.
- Regular exercise can improve the way you look and boost your self-esteem.
- Exercise can give you something positive to focus on, providing new goals and a sense of purpose.
- Involvement in a social sport helps you to be more active and meet new people.

How much exercise can help treat depression?

Physical activity lasting between 20 and 60 minutes can help to improve your psychological well-being. But even shorter bouts of moderate intensity walking (10 to 15 minutes) can significantly improve your mood.

People with depression are recommended to follow a structured and supervised exercise programme of up to three sessions per week (lasting 45 minutes to one hour), for between 10 and 12 weeks. This programme can be delivered through a referral to an exercise programme by your GP.

What is an exercise referral?

This is when your GP sends you to a fitness trainer to help you exercise. The first exercise referral schemes were set up in the 1980s and there are around 1,300 schemes now running in the UK.

Many GPs and other healthcare professionals already refer people with heart disease, diabetes, obesity and high blood pressure to these schemes. And people with mental health problems, such as depression and anxiety, can benefit from them as well.

Once your GP has referred you to an exercise scheme, you will be asked to attend an initial assessment with a qualified fitness trainer. Together you will decide what kind of exercise programme is best for you. This might include swimming or gym sessions, group classes, or even belly-dancing lessons. The programmes most often last for between three and six months, and progress is monitored by your trainer and your GP.

What types of exercise are best for treating depression?

Aerobic activities such as brisk walking, jogging, cycling, swimming and dancing tend to be the most effective for treating depression.

Resistance exercises, such as weight lifting, may be useful for helping you to build up a better self-image. And team sports can help you to start up new friendships.

If you haven't been physically active for a while, then you may need professional supervision. If your GP is unable to refer you to an exercise scheme, there are other ways for you to start exercising.

Many local authorities run walking schemes, while others offer opportunities for doing conservation work under supervision – 'green gyms'. See the Green Gyms website at www.greengym.org.uk for more information.

Staff at your local leisure centre may also be able to provide advice on how you can begin exercising safely.

What are the other benefits of exercise?

Exercising isn't just good for your mood. Your whole body will benefit from regular physical activity.

Aerobic activities such as brisk walking, jogging, cycling, swimming and dancing tend to be the most effective for treating depression

Exercise will help to:

- reduce coronary heart disease
- lower blood pressure and cholesterol levels
- protect against osteoporosis (brittle bones)
- prevent and control type 2 diabetes.

It may also help to:

- prevent stroke
- protect against bowel (colon) cancer
- reduce breast cancer risk in postmenopausal women
- reduce lung cancer risk.

- The above information is reprinted with kind permission from BUPA, excluding any accompanying illustrations, diagrams and graphs. Visit www.bupa.co.uk/health for more information or see page 41 for their address details.

© BUPA

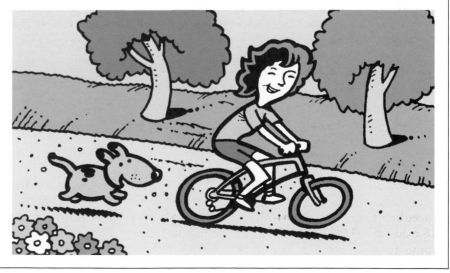

When it comes to exercise, is less more?

Six minutes of exercise a week 'is as good as six hours'

By Peter Zimonjic

Just six minutes of intense exercise a week does as much to improve a person's fitness as a regime of six hours, according to a study.

Moderately healthy men and women could cut their workouts from two hours a day, three times a week, to just two minutes a day and still achieve the same results, claim medical researchers.

Moderately healthy men and women could cut their workouts from two hours a day, three times a week, to just two minutes a day and still achieve the same results, claim researchers

The two-minute workout requires cycling furiously on a stationary bike in four 30-second bursts. Professor Martin Gibala, the author of the study, said: 'The whole excuse that "I don't have enough time to exercise" is directly challenged by these findings. This has the potential to change the way we think about keeping fit.

"We have shown that a person can get the same benefits in fitness and health in a much shorter period if they are willing to endure the discomfort of high-intensity activity.'

The study, published in this month's *Journal of Applied Physiology*, involved 23 men and women aged between 25 and 35 who were tested to see how long it took them to cycle 18.6 miles. The subjects, who all did some form of regular moderate exercise, were then given varying exercise programmes three times a week.

The first group cycled for two hours a day at a moderate pace. The second group biked harder for 10 minutes a day in 60-second bursts. The last group cycled at an intense sprint for two minutes in 30-second bursts, with four minutes of rest in between each sprint.

At the end of the two weeks each of the three groups was asked to repeat the 18.6 mile cycling test. Every subject was found to have improved to the same degree. Further tests showed that the rate at which the subjects' muscles were able to absorb oxygen also improved to the same level.

The key findings in terms of overall health showed that the two-minute workout produced the same muscle enzymes – essential for the prevention of type 2 diabetes – as riding 10 times as long. That is significant in the light of growing levels of unfitness. Obesity has trebled in Britain since 1982, leading to a rise in type 2 diabetes. The Department of Health estimates that unfit Britons cost the country £2 billion a year in the treatment of heart disease and other related illnesses.

Prof Gibala, of the health department of McMaster University in Ontario, Canada, said: 'We thought there would be benefits but we did not expect them to be this obvious. It shows how effective short intense exercise can be.'

The Sunday Telegraph put the new methods to the test by asking three employees of the Reebok Sports Club in Canary Wharf, London, to compare the workouts.

'We have shown that a person can get the same benefits in fitness and health in a much shorter period if they are willing to endure the discomfort of high-intensity activity'

Angie Du Plessis, 35, who rode for 10 minutes in 60-second sprints, said: 'It felt like I had just done an hour's run. It was more than I was used to but I feel more exhilarated because it was so intense.

'To be honest, it was not much fun and unless I was really pressed for time I would not change my exercise regime.'

Chris Mackie, 23, tried the two minutes of cycling in 30-second super-bursts and found he was exhausted very quickly. He said: 'I overworked myself well beyond what I would normally do. I can't believe it. All my energy drained so quickly.

'It was torture, really, but I was amazed at how short a time it took me to tire myself out completely. I didn't enjoy it but it felt like it worked.'

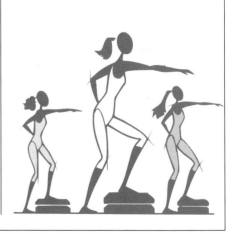

Jules Wall, 27, who rode for 45 minutes at a moderate pace, insisted that she had also received a good workout. She said: 'I am not sure I would want to go through the pain of 30-second sprints.'

Our guinea pigs were all quite fit. The authors of the study caution that anyone considering taking up cycling or running at breakneck speeds should first consult their doctor or a fitness instructor.

Just six minutes of intense exercise a week does as much to improve a person's fitness as a regime of six hours

David Crottie, a fitness expert for Reebok, was confident that the programme would be effective for anyone with the correct preparation: 'We have never tried it to this intensity before but I agree with the findings.

'Most people do not want to do it because it is so uncomfortable, but for those willing to endure the intensity it would work.'

Jonathan Edwards, the Olympic triple-jump gold medallist, said: 'Everyone seems to be short of time. If people could get fit in a much quicker period I am sure that would encourage more people to do it.

'Going for a 40-minute run is not for everybody. The idea of going and doing a short intense workout would appeal to people and help them to embrace a healthier lifestyle.'

8 June 2005

© Telegraph Group Ltd 2005

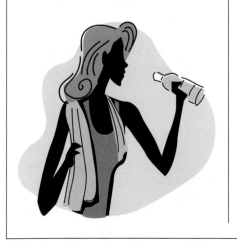

Eat well

What's a healthy diet?

Healthy eating, dieting and food fads – there are articles in nearly every newspaper and magazine. But often the messages are conflicting or misleading, and it can be hard to know what advice is nutritionally sound and accurate.

That's where the UK's national food guide comes in, known as 'The Balance of Good Health'. Eating well is all about balance and variety, and 'The Balance of Good Health' can help you achieve this. It's made up of five food groups, each group representing a different segment in the plate. Notice that these vary in size, depending on the proportions needed to make up a healthy diet.

Balancing everyday basics:
- Enjoy a variety of different foods from each food group.
- Eat regularly, including breakfast.
- Fruit and vegetables should make up one-third of the food you eat (aim for 5 or more servings per day).
- Unrefined starchy foods (e.g. bread, other cereals, pasta, rice and potatoes) should also make up about a third of your food intake.
- Eat smaller amounts of meat, fish and vegetarian alternatives, choosing lower fat options whenever possible.
- Swap high fat dairy foods, such as milk and cheese, for lower fat versions.
- Limit foods in the fatty and sugary group, and use sparingly!

For more information on food groups and healthy eating, go to the Food Standards Agency website at: www.eatwell.gov.uk

■ The above information is reprinted with kind permission from the British Dietetic Association. Visit www.bda.uk.com for more information or see page 41 for contact details.

© British Dietetic Association

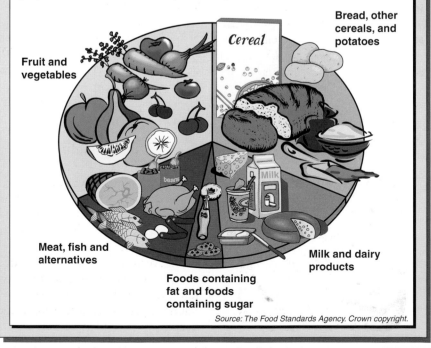

The balance of good health

The five food groups represented here vary in size, depending on the proportions needed to make up a healthy diet:

Bread, other cereals, and potatoes

Cereal

Fruit and vegetables

Meat, fish and alternatives

Foods containing fat and foods containing sugar

Milk and dairy products

Source: The Food Standards Agency. Crown copyright.

The truth about fad diets

Information from the British Dietetic Association

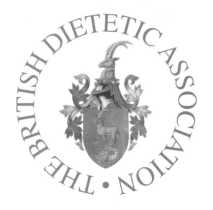

Introduction

Recent research conducted by the British Dietetic Association found that a third of people quizzed ended up heavier than their original weight only weeks after dieting. Does this sound familiar?

Part of the reason for this may be the current popularity of fad diets – the kind of regimens where you eat a very restrictive diet or an unusual combination of foods for a short period of time, lose weight quickly, but then get fed up, start eating all the wrong foods and pile the pounds back on.

To help you out of this cycle we've come up with some tips to help guide you through the maze of dietary information that surrounds us.

How to spot bad dietary advice

Stay away from diets that:

- Promise a quick fix.
- Recommend magical fat-burning effects of foods (e.g. grapefruit).
- Promote the avoidance or severe limitation of a whole food group, such as carbohydrate foods or dairy foods (and suggest large doses of vitamin and mineral supplements as a replacement).
- Promote eating mainly one type of food (e.g. cabbage soup or eggs).
- Suggest easy, rapid weight loss (more than 2lbs a week).
- Recommend eating foods only in particular combinations.
- Make claims that sound 'too good to be true'.
- Focus only on your appearance rather than on health benefits.

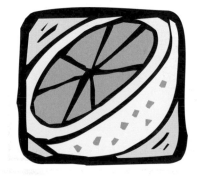

Who knows what?

Don't be fooled by the fact that many beautiful celebrities are following some of these weird and bizarre regimens. They are blessed with 'beauty' genes, and usually have armies of trainers, chefs and stylists rather than nutrition qualifications.

You should also be wary of unqualified practitioners who may be offering unproven techniques for diagnosis and treatment of nutritional problems. Be very sceptical of the following:

- Iridology
- Kinesiology
- Craniosacral therapy
- Hair mineral analysis
- Face reading
- Tongue reading
- Colonic irrigation
- Magnetic therapy.

Seek the advice of a your doctor or Registered Dietitian (RD). Registered Dietitians have recognised qualifications and will be able to give you safe, unbiased, evidence-based advice.

Basic guidelines

So what's the best advice for getting rid of the extra pounds and keeping them off? You need to think about not only the food you eat but also your lifestyle and the amount of activity you do.

You also need to think carefully about ways of changing your behaviour and developing new healthier habits if you are to lose weight and keep it off in the longer term.

Here are a few ideas to get you going

- Keep a diary and stay more aware of habits and problem areas.
- Choose lower fat foods, e.g. lean meat and lower fat dairy products.
- Watch those portion sizes!
- Fill up on vegetables and fruit as snacks and for desserts.

Don't be fooled by the fact that many beautiful celebrities are following some of these weird and bizarre regimens

- Have regular meals, starting with breakfast.
- Get active, aim for at least 30 minutes daily of moderate activity. If you can manage more than that even better – ideally aim to build up to 60 minutes a day!
- Be realistic about weight loss; aim to lose 1-2lbs (0.5-1kg) a week.

Get weight wise

And why not check out our fantastic new interactive website at: www.bdaweightwise.com designed for people of all ages and packed full of information, practical advice and support for anyone who is managing their weight.

Designed by registered dietitians and funded with a grant from the Department of Health, all the information is independent, scientifically sound, and trustworthy! And what's more – it's all free!

- The above information is reprinted with kind permission from the British Dietetic Association. Visit www.bda.uk.com for more information or see page 41 for contact details.

© British Dietetic Association

Exercise and your heart

Why is physical actvity so important for your heart?

Exactly how and why physical activity plays such an important part in preventing coronary heart disease is still the subject of research. However, it appears to act in the following ways.

Physical activity helps improve your blood cholesterol levels

Physical activity seems to raise HDL cholesterol (the 'protective' cholesterol), but does not affect LDL cholesterol levels. However, in order to maintain the benefit in HDL cholesterol, you have to make sure that you do regular physical activity.

It helps prevent blood clotting

A heart attack usually occurs when blood clots form over atheroma in the coronary arteries. Regular exercise helps to prevent blood clotting.

It helps to lower high blood pressure, and prevent high blood pressure from developing

High blood pressure is one of the four major risk factors for coronary heart disease. In 9 out of 10 people

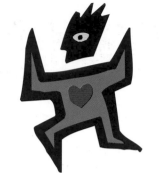

with high blood pressure there is no single underlying cause. However, unhealthy lifestyles play an important part. In particular, being overweight or obese, eating too much salt, drinking too much alcohol, and physical inactivity can all raise blood pressure.

Regular, moderate rhythmic exercise, such as walking or swimming, helps to reduce blood pressure in people with high blood pressure. This sort of exercise may also prevent high blood pressure from developing.

Physical activity helps you to maintain or reach a healthy weight

Regular physical activity plays an important part in maintaining or reaching a healthy weight. The amount of activity you do is as important as the food you eat, because being a healthy weight means balancing the energy taken into the body (the calories in your food and drink) with the energy you use up (as activity). Also, people who are obese are more likely to have high blood pressure and raised blood cholesterol levels.

It helps with diabetes

Men who have diabetes are two to three times more likely to get coronary heart disease than those without diabetes. Women with diabetes are four to five times more likely to get it.

> Being overweight or obese, eating too much salt, drinking too much alcohol, and physical inactivity can all raise blood pressure

If you already have diabetes, physical activity can help to reduce the amount of medicines or injections you need to take. Moderate, rhythmic exercise appears to reduce the risk of developing diabetes in middle-aged people, whether or not they are obese.

It helps after you have had a heart attack

Stress, depression and anxiety all appear to slow down recovery after a heart attack. There is some evidence to show that physical activity may help to relieve depression and anxiety, and therefore speed up recovery.

■ Information reprinted with kind permission from the British Heart Foundation. Visit www.bhf.org.uk for more information or see page 41 for contact details.

© British Heart Foundation

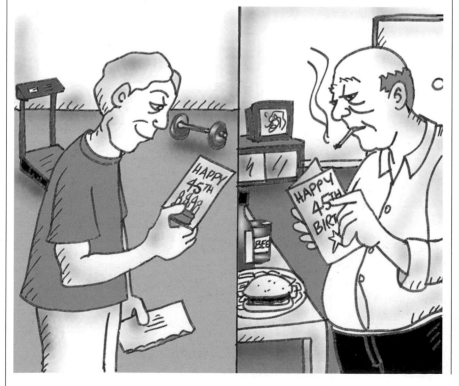

Motivation

Information from Absolute Fitness

Some people have the same burning desire to exercise as others do to taste wine, or read, or follow a football team. For others, getting their training shoes on can be a real struggle.

There is no shame in this – even fitness fanatics have days when there is nothing they would rather do than curl up in front of the telly with a bag of crisps! If you are having a hard time getting motivated, you just need to work on finding an activity that does motivate you.

Have an exercise partner. You can spur each other on and you're far more likely to get out there in the first place

A great way to ensure you are motivated is to employ a personal trainer. Not only will you be getting the very best advice from a fitness expert; the individually tailored programmes are designed specifically to keep you motivated – by making sessions enjoyable, and ultimately by ensuring you see real results.

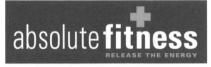

Here are a few more ideas to help you maintain motivation:

- **Have an exercise partner.** You can spur each other on and you're far more likely to get out there in the first place.
- **Vary your routines.** Doing the same exercises over and over again can quickly become dull. Mix up running, swimming, weights, tennis, hiking – the list is endless.
- **Get some good equipment.** Believe it or not, getting a new pair of running shoes or a top-of-the-range tennis racquet can really help provide some missing motivation.
- **Test your fitness regularly.** Keeping track of positive changes to weight, your resting heartbeat, or how fast you can run a mile can help give meaning to exercise and stop your motivation waning.
- **Combine exercise with leisure.** It's amazing how far you can go on a cycling machine while you are watching TV, and listening to music when you go jogging has a similar effect.

Doing the same exercises over and over again can quickly become dull

- **Don't set yourself unrealistic goals.** If you are a couple of stones overweight, don't expect to look like Brad Pitt within a few weeks. Set targets to aim for, but make them achievable – it's easy to lose motivation if you feel you are not getting anywhere.
- **Don't make weight loss your only target.** If you are losing fat but gaining heavy muscle, it can make it seem like you are not getting anywhere. Use an item of clothing that has become too tight as a reference instead – aim to fit into it in 3-6 months.

The most important thing is to choose activities that you enjoy. If you find that you are losing interest in something, think of ways to make it more fun – don't give up!

- The above information is reprinted with kind permission from Absolute Fitness. For more information, please see page 41 for contact details or visit their website at www.absolutefitness.co.uk

© Absolute Fitness

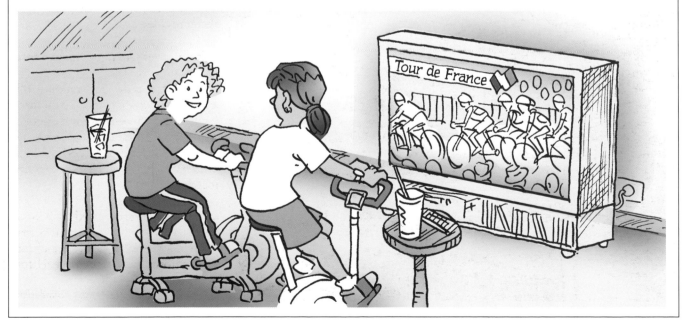

The gym

Follow TheSite's induction to the gym and you'll be a fitness freak in no time

Will the gym fix it?

The beauty of a gym workout is that you can tailor your training according to your needs. If you want to focus on developing a washboard stomach that's fine: stick to the weights room. Alternatively, you might have a broader aim, such as getting into shape with a regular cardiovascular routine, in which case head for the running machine. All gyms offer a range of different equipment, along with trained staff to help you work out how to make the most of it all. You may even find swimming pools and saunas, as well as organised classes so you can perspire with like-minded people.

Finding the right gym for you

So, you've heard from a mate that this is the only gym in town worth joining. That's great, but what if everyone shares the same opinion? A state-of-the-art rowing machine isn't much use if ten people are queuing to have a go. So ask how many members the gym has on its books, and before you sign up, make a couple of visits at the times you are most likely to be there to gauge just how busy it gets.

When you have made a shortlist, ask if they give free induction sessions. Most gyms do – and it gives you a good insight into the equipment

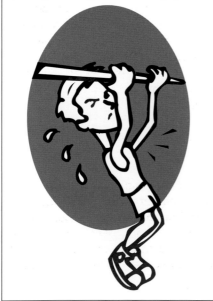

and facilities on offer. Some gyms also offer members a chance to invite a guest – ask friends at other gyms if you can go along with them for a session to get a feel of the place.

Are they registered with the Fitness Industry Association (FIA)?

The FIA is the UK's recognised body when it comes to maintaining standards in the health and fitness sector. If your gym is registered, it means they must obey a code of practice regarding safety, insurance and delivery of service. If in doubt, ask to see their plaque or certificate.

Is help at hand?

Will there be a qualified instructor on hand to show you how to work the equipment and draw up the best routine for you? There should be. An induction period is the only way to make sure you're getting the most out of the facilities, and not placing yourself in danger of death by dumb-bells.

What is your budget?

So you want to mix with celebs in Pilates classes, and have access to a private sauna once you've finished working out with your personal trainer? Hey, that's fine. This kind of thing is available, if you can afford it. According to the Fitness Industry Association, the number of gyms in the UK has rocketed by 25% since 1996, and this has broadened the range and scope of the market. The key, of course, is cost.

Gym prices can start at around twenty pounds a month, so chances are you'll find something to suit your needs. From upmarket gyms with pools and personal trainers, to everyday workout facilities with a drinks machine that's permanently out of order, the fitness world is your oyster, so work out what you can afford and seriously consider how much you'll use your membership. Also note that you'll probably have

to pay a joining fee before you start shelling out on a weekly/monthly basis, which can make it pricey to kick off.

It's estimated that almost half of all gym recruits return to the sofa within a year

---

On a tight budget? Visit your local authority sports centre and see what kind of workout facilities they have on offer. There will undoubtedly be fewer perks, but they may offer discounts to students and the unemployed, as well as off-peak membership, which is always cheaper because you are only allowed to visit at certain times.

How can I quit?

It's estimated that almost half of all gym recruits return to the sofa within a year, so it's worth checking your get-out clause before you sign up. Some require three months' written notice before you can quit, which could create financial problems if you want out because you're skint.

What do I need?

- Comfortable workout clothes. From your basic T-shirt, shorts and trainers, to expensive vests, headbands, and, naturally, all manner of figure-hugging Lycra wear.
- An income. Most gyms are membership only, often at around £30 a month. When you cost in the joining fee, this isn't the kind of path to fitness that should be taken if you're not committed (and cash-ready).

■ The above information is reprinted with kind permission from TheSite.org. Visit www.thesite.org for more information.

© TheSite.org

Compulsive exercise

Information from KidsHealth

Rachel and her cheerleading team practise three to five times a week. Rachel feels a lot of pressure to keep her weight down – as head cheerleader, she wants to set an example to the team. So she adds extra daily workouts to her regimen. But lately, Rachel has been feeling worn out, and she has a hard time just making it through a regular team practice.

You may think you can't get too much of a good thing, but in the case of exercise, a healthy activity can sometimes turn into an unhealthy compulsion. Rachel is a good example of how an overemphasis on physical fitness or weight control can become unhealthy. Read on to find out more about compulsive exercise and its effects.

Too much of a good thing?

We all know the benefits of exercise, and it seems that everywhere we turn, we hear that we should exercise more. The right kind of exercise does many great things for your body and soul: it can strengthen your heart and muscles, lower your body fat, and reduce your risk of many diseases.

Many teens who play sports have higher self-esteem than their less active pals, and exercise can even

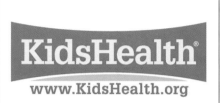

www.KidsHealth.org

help keep the blues at bay because of the endorphin rush it can cause. Endorphins are naturally produced chemicals that affect your sensory perception. These chemicals are released in your body during and after a workout and they go a long way in helping to control stress.

So how can something with so many benefits have the potential to cause harm?

Lots of people start working out because it's fun or it makes them feel good, but exercise can become a compulsive habit when it is done for the wrong reasons.

Some people start exercising with weight loss as their main goal. Although exercise is part of a safe and healthy way to control weight, many people may have unrealistic expectations. We are bombarded with images from advertisers of the ideal body: young and thin for women; strong and muscular for men.

To try to reach these unreasonable ideals, people may turn to diets, and, for some, this may develop into eating disorders such as anorexia and bulimia. And some people who grow frustrated with the results from diets alone may overexercise to speed up weight loss.

Lots of people start working out because it's fun or it makes them feel good, but exercise can become a compulsive habit when it is done for the wrong reasons

---

Some athletes may also think that repeated exercise will help them to win an important game. Like Rachel, they add extra workouts to those regularly scheduled with their teams without consulting their coaches or trainers. The pressure to succeed may also lead these people to exercise more than is healthy. The body needs activity but it also needs rest. Over-exercising can lead to injuries like fractures and muscle strains.

Are you a healthy exerciser?

Fitness experts recommend that teens do at least 60 minutes of moderate to vigorous physical activity every day. Most young people exercise much less than this recommended amount (which can be a problem for different reasons), but some – such as athletes – do more.

Experts say that repeatedly exercising beyond the requirements for good health is an indicator of compulsive behaviour. Some people need more than the average amount of exercise, of course – such as athletes in training for a big event. But several workouts a day, every day, when a person is not in training is a sign that the person is probably overdoing it.

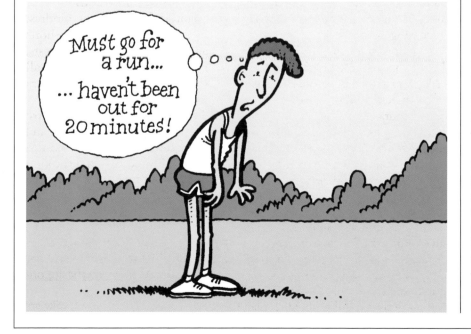

Must go for a run... ...haven't been out for 20 minutes!

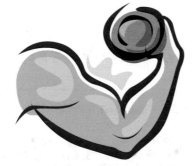

People who are exercise dependent also go to extremes to fit activity into their lives. If you put workouts ahead of friends, homework, and other responsibilities, you may be developing a dependence on exercise.

> *If you put workouts ahead of friends, homework, and other responsibilities, you may be developing a dependence on exercise*

If you are concerned about your own exercise habits or a friend's, ask yourself the following questions. Do you:

- force yourself to exercise, even if you don't feel well?
- prefer to exercise rather than being with friends?
- become very upset if you miss a workout?
- base the amount you exercise on how much you eat?
- have trouble sitting still because you think you're not burning calories?
- worry that you'll gain weight if you skip exercising for a day?

If the answer to any of these questions is yes, you or your friend may have a problem. What should you do?

How to get help
The first thing you should do if you suspect that you are a compulsive exerciser is get help. Talk to your parents, doctor, a teacher or counsellor, a coach, or another trusted adult. Compulsive exercise, especially when it is combined with an eating disorder, can cause serious and permanent health problems, and, in extreme cases, death.

Because compulsive exercise is closely related to eating disorders, help can be found at community agencies specifically set up to deal with anorexia, bulimia, and other eating problems. Your school's health or physical education department may also have support programmes and nutrition advice available. Ask

your teacher, coach, or counsellor to recommend local organisations that may be able to help.

You should also schedule a checkup with a doctor. Because our bodies go through so many important developments during the teen years, guys and girls who have compulsive exercise problems need to see a doctor to make sure they are developing normally. This is especially true if the person also has an eating disorder. Female athlete triad, a condition that affects girls who overexercise and restrict their eating because of their sports, can cause a girl to stop having her period. Medical help is necessary to resolve the physical problems associated with overexercising before they cause long-term damage to the body.

Make a positive change
Changes in activity of any kind – eating or sleeping, for example – can often be a sign that something else is wrong in your life. Girls and guys who exercise compulsively may have a distorted body image and low self-esteem. They may see themselves as overweight or out of shape even when they are actually a healthy weight.

Compulsive exercisers need to get professional help for the reasons described above. But there are also some things that you can do to help you take charge again:

- Work on changing your daily self-talk. When you look in the mirror, make sure you find at least one good thing to say about yourself. Be more aware of your positive attributes.
- When you exercise, focus on the positive, mood-boosting qualities.
- Give yourself a break. Listen to your body and give yourself a day of rest after a hard workout.
- Control your weight by exercising and eating moderate portions of healthy foods. Don't try to change your body into an unrealistically lean shape. Talk with your doctor, dietitian, coach, athletic trainer, or other adult about what a healthy body weight is for you and how to develop healthy eating and exercise habits.

Exercise and sports are supposed to be fun and keep you healthy. Working out in moderation will do both.

- This information was provided by KidsHealth, one of the largest resources online for medically reviewed health information for parents, kids and teens. For more articles like this one, visit their websites at www.teenshealth.org or www.kidshealth.org

© 1995-2005. *The Nemours Foundation*

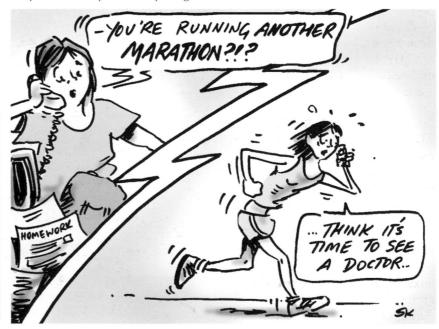

The benefits of exercise

Information from Absolute Fitness

Physical benefits

It's a question that has gone through everyone's mind from time to time – why bother? Wouldn't I be happier lifting a pint instead of this dumbbell? Why am I running in the rain instead of (insert your favourite pastime here) – am I mad?!

But there's a good reason why you are putting yourself through your paces. In fact, there are hundreds of good reasons, and we all know what they are – we just need reminding from time to time.

One of the biggest killers of the modern age is lack of exercise. It's as simple as that. By taking even moderate exercise on a regular basis our immune system is strengthened – and we cut the risk of heart disease, stroke, blood vessel disorders, thrombosis, angina; the list goes on. The key word here is regular: all exercise is good, but regular moderate exercise has a greater effect on your overall health than occasional bursts of lung-busting activity. In short, be as active as you can, as often as possible – and KEEP IT GOING!!!

Life just seems much easier when you are fit – and it's not just the body that benefits from exercise. Exercise triggers chemical changes in the brain that can have a powerful and positive effect on mental health.

The ability to deal with the daily demands of hard work and play more effectively is one of the most underestimated side effects of fitness – and one of the best!

Psychological benefits

The psychological benefits of regular exercise can be as significant as the physical. Some, such as better self-esteem, come as an indirect result of exercise and are fairly subjective.

Others are a direct consequence of chemical activity triggered by physical exertion – for example, people suffering from depression or anxiety are often 'prescribed' exercise. Brain chemicals released during exercise, such as serotonin,

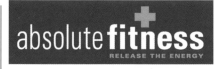

dopamine, norepinephrine, and endorphins, are known to have strong effects on mood, helping reduce feelings of anxiety, stress and depression, while also helping to strengthen your immune system.

Twenty different types of endorphin have been discovered in the nervous system, and the beta-endorphins secreted during exercise have the most powerful effect. Sometimes described as 'runners' high', the release of beta-endorphins reduces pain (the reason why running becomes easier after about 20 minutes) and stimulates feelings of euphoria – which is why so many people feel invigorated and enthusiastic after exercise.

Other psychological side effects of exercise include:

- Improved self-esteem and greater sense of self-reliance and self-confidence.
- Improved mental alertness, perception and information processing.
- Increased perceptions of acceptance by others.
- Decreased overall feelings of stress and tension.

- Reduced frustration with daily problems, and a more constructive response to disappointments and failures.

These psychological benefits can be just as important as the more obvious physical ones; most of us exercise in the first place because we are unhappy about something, whether it is that spare tyre, worries about general health, or just being sick of feeling tired and unfit.

By taking even moderate exercise on a regular basis our immune system is strengthened

If you are feeling like a couch potato, or you are finding stress and worry is becoming a problem, get out there and exercise! The hardest part by far is that initial step, when it can feel like exercise is the last thing in the world that will cheer you up: try to remember that exercise is one of the very best ways to do just that.

- The above information is reprinted with kind permission from Absolute Fitness. For more information, see page 41 for contact details or visit www.absolutefitness.co.uk

© Absolute Fitness

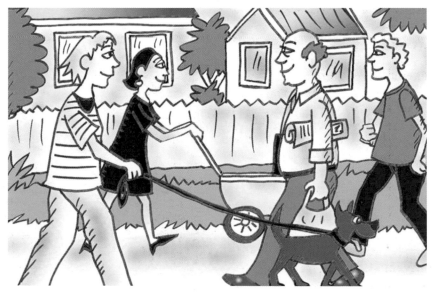

■ Only 10 per cent of young people get the one hour a day of physical activity that ministers, health experts and scientists say is necessary. (page 1)

■ The amount of time kids spend watching televison is a key factor in childhood obesity, a new study suggests. (page 2)

■ Globally more than 1 billion adults are overweight and 300 million adults are obese. Approximately 17.6 million children are overweight worldwide. (page 2)

■ The percentage of children aged 2 to 10 who were overweight (including those who were obese) rose from 22.7% in 1995 to 27.7% in 2003. (page 3)

■ While in general, three-quarters (75%) of parents with children under 16 claim that they try to ensure their kids eat a healthy diet, only just over half (54%) say that they try to actually educate their children about healthy eating. (page 4)

■ Many obese teenagers could face heart attacks in their 40s, according to the medical director of the British Heart Foundation. (page 5)

■ 40-69% of children over the age of six spend less than the recommended minimum of one hour a day doing moderate intensity physical activity. (page 7)

■ Studies show that breastfeeding a baby, even if only for a short period of time, may reduce the risk of obesity in later life. (page 8)

■ People gain weight when the body takes in more calories than it burns off. Those extra calories are stored as fat. (page 9)

■ The BMI is a tool for indicating weight status in adults. It is a measure of weight for height. (page 11)

■ 48% of all British adults are 'fed up with being told what to eat by "do-gooders" on healthy eating campaigns'. (page 13)

■ 47% of men were classed overweight in 2001, compared to 33% of females. (page 14)

■ The majority of UK adults are unaware that having a large waist (abdominal obesity) is a root cause of diabetes and heart disease, according to a new survey. (page 15)

■ Being a little overweight is good for you, a study suggests. But being stick-thin increases the risk of death, according to the research. (page 15)

■ It is harder to find a job if you are overweight than if you are slim according to a survey of personnel officers. (page 17)

■ It's estimated that, in England and Wales, 18m working days a year are lost to obesity. (page 17)

■ Almost three-quarters of Scots blamed a poor diet at work for weight gain. (page 18)

■ It is estimated that about 36% of deaths from coronary heart disease in men and 38% of deaths in women are due to lack of physical activity. (page 20)

■ Physical activity improves both your physical and mental health. It is one of the most important factors in maintaining a good quality of life. (page 21)

■ Experts recommend that adults get more than 60 minutes of moderate to vigorous physical activity each day. (page 22)

■ Different authorities have differing opinions on what makes someone 'fit'. The bottom line is this: if you're physically fit, you can do your chosen form of exercise without ending up completely exhausted. (page 24)

■ With cars on most driveways and the decline in the number of physically active jobs, 70% of the adult population is sufficiently inactive to be classed as 'sedentary'. (page 25)

■ Exercise may be just as effective at treating depression as antidepressant medicines, according to a report from the Mental Health Foundation. (page 29)

■ Just six minutes of intense exercise a week does as much to improve a person's fitness as a regime of six hours, according to a study. (page 31)

■ A heart attack usually occurs when blood clots form over atheroma in the coronary arteries. Regular exercise helps to prevent blood clotting. (page 34)

■ It's estimated that almost half of all gym recruits return to the sofa within a year. (page 36)

■ Endorphins are naturally produced chemicals that affect your sensory perception. These chemicals are released in your body during and after a workout and they go a long way in helping to control stress. (page 37)

■ Regular moderate exercise has a greater effect on your overall health than occasional hours of lung-busting activity. (page 39)

ADDITIONAL RESOURCES

You might like to contact the following organisations for further information. Due to the increasing cost of postage, many organisations cannot respond to enquiries unless they receive a stamped, addressed envelope.

Absolute Fitness
1a Vincent House
Vincent Square
LONDON
SW1P 2NB
Tel: 020 7834 0000
Fax: 020 7834 0815
Email: info@absolutefitness.co.uk
Website:
www.absolutefitness.co.uk
Kathryn Freeland, founder of Absolute Fitness, created the Absolute Standard™ to assure you of the best possible service. Established in 1997 Absolute Fitness is now recognised as the foremost mobile personal training company in London.

Association for the Study of Obesity (ASO)
Eversheds House
70 Great Bridgewater Street
MANCHESTER
M1 5ES
Tel: 020 8503 2042
Fax: 020 8503 2442
Website: www.aso.org.uk
A UK company limited by guarantee; registered in England and Wales No. 4796449; registered charity No. 1100648. The ASO promotes research into the causes, prevention and treatment of obesity, encourages action to reduce the prevalence of obesity, and facilitates contact between individuals and organisations interested in weight regulation.

British Dietetic Association
5th Floor, Charles House
148/9 Great Charles Street,
Queensway
BIRMINGHAM
B3 3HT
Tel: 0121 200 8080
Fax: 0121 200 8081
Email: info@bda.uk.com
Websites: www.bda.uk.com
www.bdaweightwise.com/bda/
The British Dietetic Association, established in 1936, is the professional association for dietitians. The association was established to advance the science and practice of dietetics and associated subjects, promote training and education in the science and practice of dietetics and associated subjects and regulate the relations between dietitians and their employer through the BDA Trade Union.

British Heart Foundation (BHF)
14 Fitzhardinge Street
LONDON
W1H 4DH
Tel: 020 7935 0185
Fax: 020 7486 5820
Email: internet@bhf.org.uk
www.bhf.org.uk
The aim of the British Heart Foundation is to play a leading role in the fight against heart disease and prevent death by ways including educating the public and health professionals about heart disease, its prevention and treament.

BUPA
Bupa House
15-19 Bloomsbury Way
LONDON
WC1A 2BA
Tel: 020 7656 2055
020 7656 2716
botte@bupa.com
www.bupa.co.uk

KidsHealth
The Nemours Foundation
1600 Rockland Road
Wilmington, DE 19803
USA
Tel: +1 302 651 4046
Email: info@KidsHealth.org
www.kidshealth.org
KidsHealth is the largest and most visited site on the Web providing doctor-approved health information about children from before birth through adolescence. Created by The Nemours Foundation's Center for Children's Health Media.

National Heart Forum
Tavistock House South
Tavistock Square
LONDON
WC1H 9LG
Tel: 020 7383 7638
Fax: 020 7387 2799
Email:
webenquiry@heartforum.org.uk
Website: www.heartforum.org.uk

National Obesity Forum
PO Box 6625
NOTTINGHAM
NG2 5PA
Tel: 0115 8462109
Fax: 0115 8462109
Email:
info@nationalobesityforum.org.uk
Website:
www.nationalobesityforum.org.uk
The National Obesity Forum was established in May 2000 to raise awareness of the growing impact of obesity and overweight on our patients and our National Health Service. Membership is open to all healthcare professionals and is free. Through our activities we aim to improve the delivery of best practice in the management of obesity. The National Obesity Forum is an independent medical organisation.

Weight Concern
Brook House
2-16 Torrington Place
LONDON
WC1E 7HN
Tel: 020 7679 66 36
Fax: 020 7813 2848
Email:
enquiries@weightconcern.com
Website: www.weightconcern.com
Weight Concern is a registered charity, set up in 1997 to tackle the rising problem of obesity in the United Kingdom.
The charity, which won the Best New Charity of the Year Award in 2002, works to address both the physical and psychological health needs of overweight people.

INDEX

abdominal obesity, health risks 11, 15
absenteeism and obesity 17
activity *see* exercise
advertisement of junk food, effect on childhood obesity 2
aerobic exercise 22
affluence, relationship with obesity 12
ageing, benefits of exercise 22
alcohol as food weakness 14
amenorrhoea 23
Atkins diet, effect on eating habits 14

Balance of Good Health food guide 32
balanced diet *see* healthy eating
blood cholesterol and exercise 34
blood pressure and exercise 34
body mass index (BMI) 9, 11, 31

calorie intake recording 31
cardio-respiratory endurance 24
childhood obesity 1-5, 6, 7-8, 12
    importance of exercise 6
    and television 2
children
    diet 4-5, 8
    need for exercise 1, 6, 8
    and sport safety 28
    see also childhood obesity
cholesterol and exercise 34
compulsive exercise 37-8
coronary heart disease 19-20
costs
    gym membership 36
    to health service of coronary heart disease 20
cross training 28

deaths from coronary heart disease 19
defensive eating 32
depression
    and exercise 29-30
    and obesity 10
diabetes
    benefits of exercise 34
    obesity as risk factor 15
diet
    children's 4-5, 8
    and coronary heart disease 20

healthy *see* healthy eating
    and weight maintenance 31-2
dieting 33
discomfort after exercise 27

eating disorders and compulsive exercise 38
eating habits *see* diet; healthy eating
emotional benefits of exercise 22
emotional factors in obesity 9
emotional significance of food 8
employment and obesity 17
enjoying exercise 31, 35
exercise 10, 21-30, 34-9
    barriers to 25
    benefits 21, 22-3, 25, 30
    children 1, 6, 8
    and depression 29-30
    and the heart 34
    lack of *see* inactivity
    motivation for 26, 35
    recommended amounts 22-3, 25-6, 27, 31, 37
        children 1
    and weight reduction 31
exercise referral 30

fad diets 33
families and obesity 9
fat in diet 14, 20
female athlete triad 23, 38
fitness 21, 24, 26, 27-8
    benefits of walking 39
    motivation 35
    see also exercise
Fitness Industry Association (FIA) 36
flexibility training 23
food weaknesses, Britain 13-14

genes and obesity 9
girls, problems of overexercise 23, 28
gyms 36

health benefits
    physical activity 21, 22-3, 25, 29-30, 34
    walking 39
health risks
    of obesity 5, 7, 10

ACKNOWLEDGEMENTS

The publisher is grateful for permission to reproduce the following material.

While every care has been taken to trace and acknowledge copyright, the publisher tenders its apology for any accidental infringement or where copyright has proved untraceable. The publisher would be pleased to come to a suitable arrangement in any such case with the rightful owner.

Chapter One: Our Fitness Problem

90% of children set to be couch potatoes, © Guardian Newspapers Ltd 2005, *TV link to obese children*, © Which?, *How many people are obese?*, © Weight Concern, *Obesity among children under 11*, © Crown copyright is reproduced with the permission of Her Majesty's Stationery Office, *Childhood obesity*, © Mintel, *Children's diets*, © Weight Loss Resources, *Call for Jamie Oliver of the gym*, © Guardian Newspapers Ltd 2005, *Avoiding childhood obesity*, © BUPA, *Obesity*, © 1995-2005. The Nemours Foundation, *Obesity: the scale of the problem*, © Association for the Study of Obesity, *Half of Britain fed up with healthy eating do-gooders!*, © Mintel, *48 million adults unaware of health time bomb*, © National Obesity Forum, *Being overweight is good for your health, says study*, © 2005 Associated Newspapers Ltd, *The question*, © Guardian Newspapers Ltd 2005, *Being overweight can impede job prospects*, © Surgery Door, *Snacking at work blamed for unfit employees*, © The Scotsman 2005, *Facts about coronary heart disease*, © National Heart Forum.

Chapter Two: Getting Fit

Get active!, © British Heart Foundation, *Why exercise is wise*, © 1995-2005. The Nemours Foundation, *Getting fit*, © TheSite.org, *Physical activity*, © BUPA, *Physical exercise*, © Crown copyright is reproduced with the permission of Her Majesty's Stationery Office, *Student fitness*, © TheSite.org, *Exercise beats the blues*, © BUPA, *When it comes to exercise, is less more?*, © Telegraph Group Ltd 2005, *Eat well*, © British Dietetic Association, *The truth about fad diets*, © British Dietetic Association, *Exercise and your heart*, © British Heart Foundation, *Motivation*, © Absolute Fitness, *The gym*, © TheSite.org, *Compulsive exercise*, © 1995-2005. The Nemours Foundation, *The benefits of exercise*, © Absolute Fitness.

Photographs and illustrations:

Pages 1, 34, 39: Bev Aisbett; pages 12, 28, 30, 37: Don Hatcher; pages 13, 24: Pumpkin House; pages 16, 20, 27, 38: Simon Kneebone; pages 18, 26, 29, 35: Angelo Madrid.

Craig Donnellan
Cambridge
January, 2006